LUPUS DIET COOKBOOK

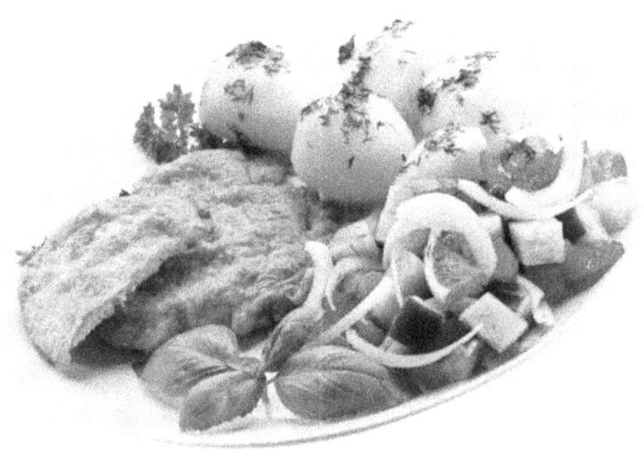

Recipes for Ultra-Nourishing Foods That Can Help Reverse Autoimmune Diseases

Joan G. Milone

Copyright © 2024 by Joan G. Milone

All rights reserved.

No part of this book may be reproduced, stored in a retrieval system, or transmitted in any form or by any means, electronic, mechanical, photocopying, recording, or otherwise, without prior written permission of the copyright owner.

This book is written as a source of information only. The information contained in this book is provided in good faith and is believed to be accurate and reliable as of the date of publication. The author does not assume any responsibility for any errors or omissions that may appear.

Scan To Access More Amazing Cookbooks from Joan

Table of Content

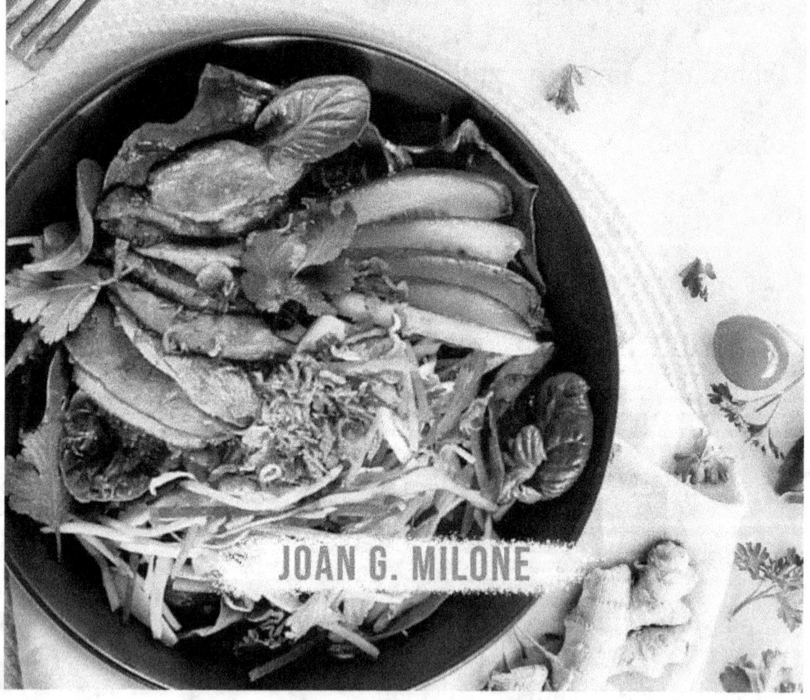
LUPUS
DIET COOKBOOK
Recipes for Ultra-Nourishing Foods That Can
Help Reverse Autoimmune Diseases
JOAN G. MILONE

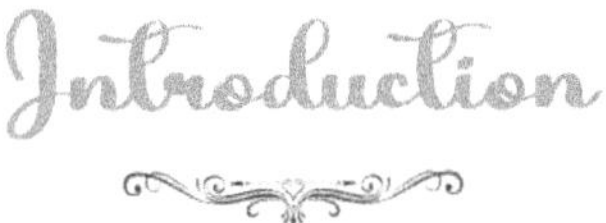

Introduction

Step into my kitchen, a sanctuary where the perfume of herbs and the soothing hum of the stove tell the narrative of my lupus fights. I'm not only an author and a dietitian; I've witnessed the quiet battles and victories that emerge inside the fabric of a chronic disease. So, please join me in the world I've created within the pages of "Lupus Cookbook for Beginners."

This cookbook is more than simply a collection of recipes; it's a journal of my journey, in which every spoonful of deliciousness represented a little win over the hardships of lupus. Each page flipped represents a shared experience, a bond formed by the alchemy of ingredients and the warmth of a shared table.

So, imagine waking up with me to the brilliant colors of a Tropical Sunrise Smoothie Bowl—a rush of energy to get our day started. Let's linger over a Mediterranean Chickpea Salad Bowl as we explore Lively Lunches, where the tastes take us to sunshine afternoons filled with laughter. And when the day comes to a close, join me in relishing the Lemon Herb Baked Chicken—a dish that embodies perseverance, garnished with delight.

This cookbook results from our discourse, a heart-to-heart in which lupus is the only background music to our gastronomic adventure. These aren't just recipes; they're whispers of encouragement and shared memories, from Breakfast Bliss to Salads and Soups, Poultry and Meat to Basics and Dressings.

So, my fellow lupus fighters, take up a chair and let's flip these pages together. We're not just cooking in "Lupus Cookbook," but also creating a story about strength, sustenance, and celebrating life. Welcome to my kitchen, where every dish has a tale to tell.

Understanding Lupus: A Brief Overview

Consider your immune system your body's defender, a diligent protector against intruders. Consider it temporarily losing its way and turning against its team; that's lupus.

Lupus is the unanticipated plot twist in your life's tale. It's an autoimmune condition in which the immune system becomes confused instead of praising the good guys, attacking healthy tissues and creating havoc. Consider it a case of mistaken identification on a tiny scale.

Lupus is notorious for being unpredictable. It does not adhere to a script. It might be testing your joints one day, making them feel like they've run a marathon overnight. The next thing you know, it's protesting your skin and leaving you with a nice rash as its manifesto.

The catch is that lupus does not discriminate. It might have varied effects on different people. Some have minor joint discomfort and weariness, while others experience a full-fledged symphony of symptoms ranging from renal problems to cardiac troubles.

Let us now discuss the well-known causes that might rouse lupus from its hibernation. Stress, lack of sleep, and even too much sun can increase the intensity of a lupus flare. It's like putting it in the limelight when all you want is peace and quiet.

Understanding lupus is similar to interpreting a complicated character in a novel: you come to know it piece by piece, and there's always more behind the surface. While there is no cure, controlling lupus is typically a dance, including medicine, self-care, and listening to your body's messages.

So, welcome to the complicated world of lupus, where we will negotiate the twists and turns together. It's not always easy, but comprehending this situation is the first step toward flipping the page to a new chapter in your tale, one in which you're the resilient protagonist.

The Role of Nutrition in Lupus Management

Okay, let's talk about the hero in our lupus management toolbox: nutrition. Consider it your lupus companion, ready to assist you in your fight against the disease.

Consider your body a well-tuned machine, with you as the fuel. When you have lupus, this fuel becomes even more important. It's like giving your body the tools to fix itself and keep the lupus at bay.

So, what's the strategy? First and foremost, we have antioxidants, the hidden heroes. Consider them a barrier that shields your cells from the oxidative damage induced by lupus. Your antioxidant army consists of berries, leafy greens, and bright vegetables.

Omega-3 fatty acids are the peacekeepers on the squad. They are found in fatty fish such as salmon, chia seeds, and walnuts and assist in reducing inflammation, which is equivalent to telling lupus, "Hey, let's keep things cool around here."

Let us now discuss the ultimate strategy: a balanced plate. Consider it a team gathering in which everyone brings their A-game. You've got your protein sources - the builders, whole grains and carbohydrates - the energy boosters, and healthy fats - the lifeblood. They work together to form a symphony that keeps your body humming smoothly.

The storyline twist is that individual participants may have preferences. Some lupus patients find solace in a Mediterranean-style diet emphasizing olive oil, seafood, and vegetables. Others swear by turmeric, ginger, and green tea's anti-inflammatory properties.

Hydration is now the unsung hero. Consider it the backstage team that keeps things working smoothly behind the scenes. Water flushes away pollutants and keeps your cells hydrated, assisting your body's everyday performance.

Don't forget about portion management - it's like having a well-balanced cast. Too much of a good thing isn't necessarily a good thing. So it's a matter of finding that sweet spot where you're fueling your body without overburdening it.

You are not alone on this dietary quest. It's not about limiting but about empowering. Consider it like constructing a menu tailored to your body's tastes, a blueprint for a robust you. So, sit at the nutrition table and create a plan that works for your lupus narrative - one mouthful at a time.

A Key Nutrients for Lupus Warriors

Omega-3 Fatty Acids are the first in line; they are the peacekeepers in the body's internal conflict. Think of them as the level-headed negotiators who maintain order and reduce tension. These superfoods may be found in walnuts, flaxseeds, and fatty seafood like salmon. They act as a comforting salve for the inflammatory blues in your body.

Let me introduce you to the Antioxidants - the powerful barriers that safeguard your cells from the damage produced by oxidative stress, which acts as a villain attempting to disturb the balance. Fill on berries, leafy greens, and vibrant vegetables to strengthen your immune system. Consider antioxidants as your defense team is prepared to face any challenge that lupus may present.

In this story, the unsung heroes are vitamins and minerals. The sunshine vitamin, vitamin D, helps maintain the health of your bones and immune system, functioning as a mild guide to assist your body in mounting a defense. The building block of strength, calcium, keeps your bones strong.

Next is vitamin B12, which is present in dairy, meat, and fish and is your energy ally. It is your constant companion when lupus attempts to play the tired card. Remember iron, too; it's an oxygen transporter that helps your body obtain energy and may be found in spinach, beans, and lean meats.

See these nutrients as the vivid brushstrokes on a beautiful canvas that is your plate. Making a masterpiece that strengthens your body's resistance is more important than imposing restrictions. Thus, let's honor the nutritional Avengers and make sure they take center stage in your lupus narrative—a tale of vigor, health, and well-being.

Breakfast Bliss: Kickstarting Your Day

Here, we create a symphony of tastes and nutrients out of your mornings in "Breakfast Bliss: Kickstarting Your Day," the dawn of your day. We'll explore colorful smoothie bowls, filling quinoa porridge, and nutrient-dense wraps. Envision your kitchen as a blank canvas, with every breakfast meal serving as an energetic brushstroke that sets the tone for a day when lupus takes a backseat. Let's go on a delectable voyage that brightens your day and strengthens your fortitude in the lupus journey, starting with cool smoothies and ending with cozy porridges. Breakfast, but with a dash of well-being and a sprinkling of delight.

Tropical Sunrise Smoothie Bowl

Ingredients:

- One cup of frozen mango chunks
- Half a cup of frozen pineapple chunks
- One ripe banana
- Half a cup of Greek yogurt
- One spoonful of chia seeds
- Flakes of coconut (for garnish)

Preparation:

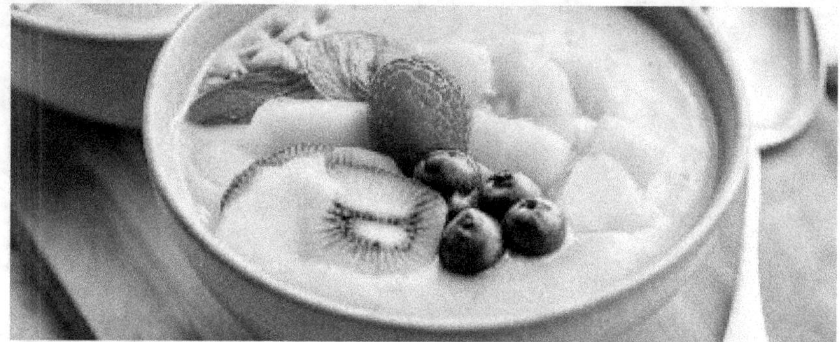

1. Smoothly blend frozen mango, banana, pineapple, and Greek yogurt.
2. Transfer the blended drink to a bowl.
3. Add chia seeds on top and coconut flakes on top.

Nutritional Value:

- Rich in antioxidants from pineapple and mango and high in vitamin C (around 80% of the recommended daily intake).
- Probiotics and protein are added by Greek yogurt (around 15% of daily value).
- Chia seeds include fiber and omega-3 fatty acids (10% of daily value).

Cooking Period: Five minutes

Quinoa and Berry Breakfast Parfait

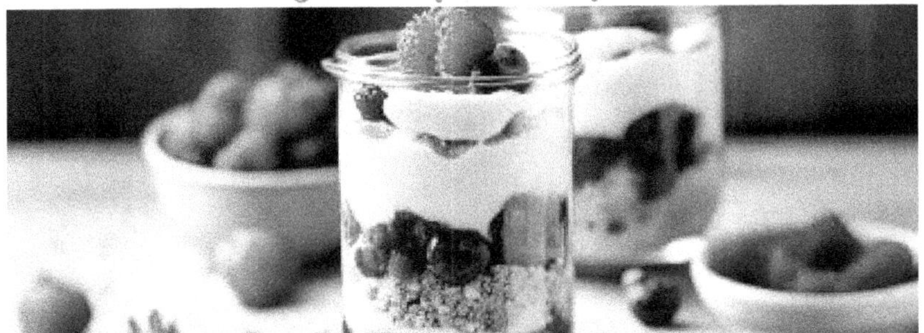

Ingredients:

- One cup of cooked quinoa
- Strawberries, blueberries, and raspberries are mixed berries.
- Greek yogurt
- Honey is optional.
- Slices of almonds (for garnish)

Preparation:

1. Arrange cooked quinoa, Greek yogurt, and mixed berries in a glass or dish.
2. Iterate through the levels.
3. Spread honey over it and arrange almond pieces on top.

Nutritional Value:

- Protein and fiber (around 15% of the daily value) are provided by quinoa.

- Antioxidants are abundant in berries (around 25% of the daily value).

- Probiotics and protein are provided by Greek yogurt (15 percent of the daily recommended amount).

- Almond slices include vitamin E (about 10% of the daily intake) and good lipids.

Cooking Period: 15 minutes (to prepare the quinoa).

Spinach and Feta Breakfast Wrap

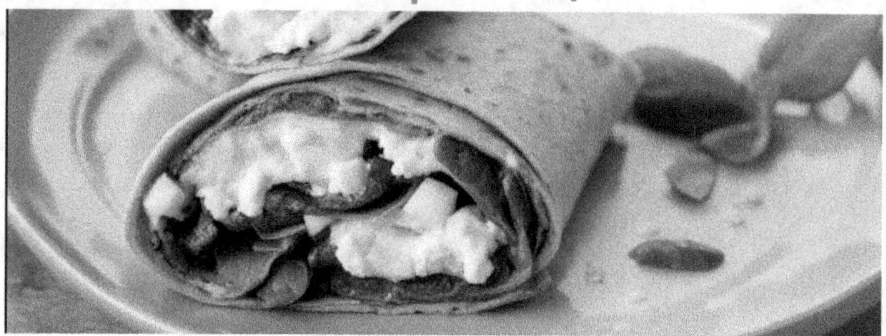

Ingredients:

- Whole-grain wrap
- Eggs scrambled
- Fried spinach

- Feta crumbles
- Cherry tomatoes are optional.

Preparation:

1. Pour scrambled eggs into a whole grain wrapper.
2. Add the crumbled feta and the sautéed spinach.
3. Add sliced cherry tomatoes, if desired.

4. If necessary, secure the wrap with a toothpick after rolling it up.

Nutritional Value:

- Eggs scrambled provide important minerals and protein (around 20% of daily intake).

- Vitamins and iron are included in spinach (15 percent of the daily value).

- 10% of the dietary value of feta comes from taste and calcium.

Cooking Period: Ten minutes

Blueberry Almond Overnight Oats

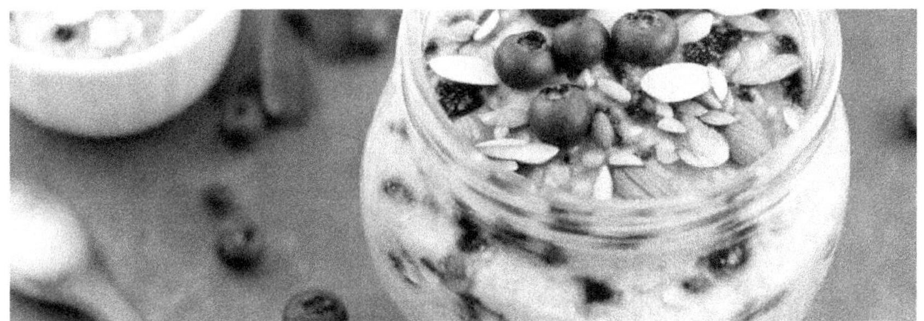

Ingredients:

- Oats rolled
- Almond milk
- Berries
- Slices of almonds
- Honey is optional.

Preparation:

1. Rolling oats, almond milk, and fresh blueberries should all be combined in a container.

2. Once combined, chill for the entire night.

3. Sprinkle almond pieces on top and, if preferred, sprinkle with honey in the morning.

Nutritional Value:

- Rolled oats offer fiber and important minerals (15 percent of daily value).

- Antioxidants are abundant in blueberries (20% of daily value).

- Almond slices include vitamin E (about 10% of the daily intake) and good lipids.

Cooking Period: Five minutes (the previous evening's preparation)

Avocado and Smoked Salmon Breakfast Toast

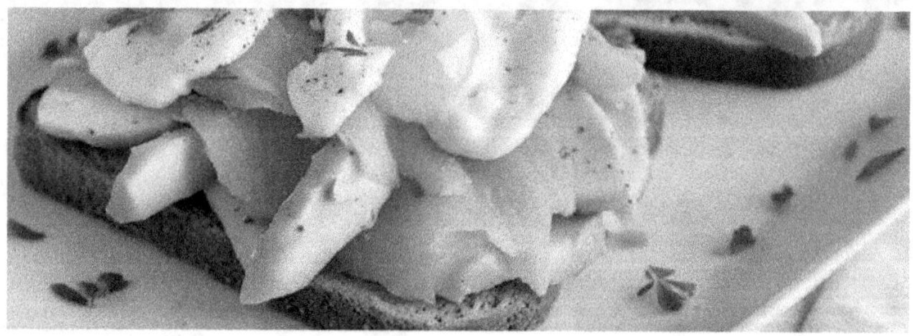

Ingredients:

- Whole-grain toast
- Mashed avocado
- Smoked salmon
- Dill Capers (optional)

Preparation:

1. To taste, toast whole grain bread.

2. Toast should be topped with mashed avocado.

3. If preferred, garnish with capers, smoked salmon, and dill.

Nutrition Value:

- Toast made from whole grains offers fiber and important nutrients (around 15% of the daily intake).

- Avocado provides vitamins and good fats (10% of daily value).

- Omega-3 fatty acids and protein are abundant in smoked salmon (20% of daily value).

Cooking Period: Five minutes

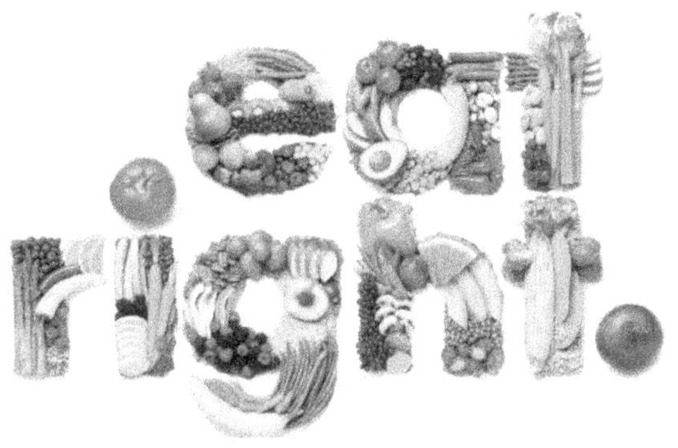

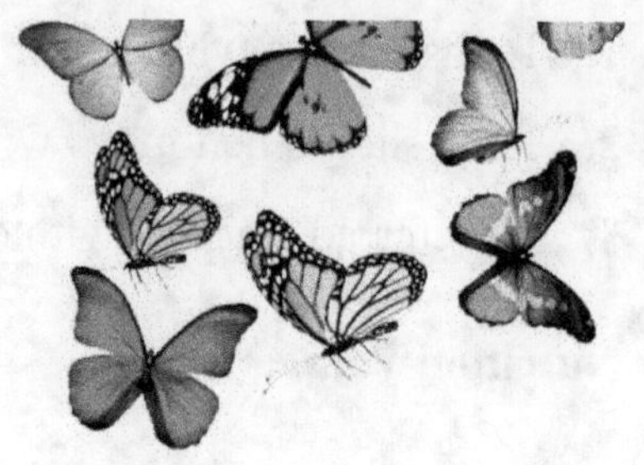

Hi there, wonderful soul! It's not easy to have lupus, but remember that you are an example of resilience, not just someone who endures. Your unshakeable courage and great strength are demonstrated by the challenges you confront every day. Lupus is only one chapter in your life; it doesn't define you. Accept the warrior that is inside you; your strength is greater than anything this illness can provide.

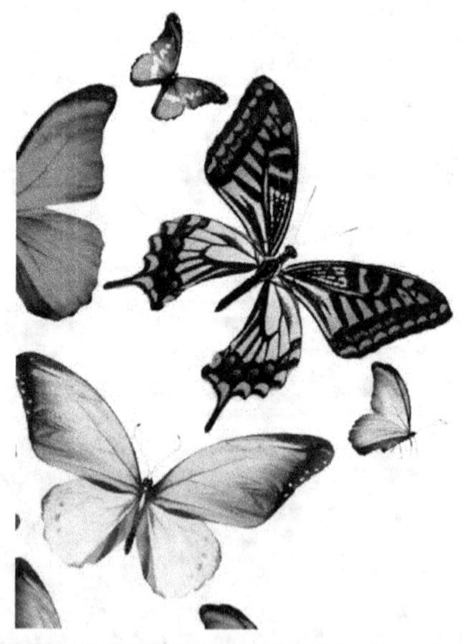

Lively Lunches: Fueling Midday

Introducing "Lively Lunches: Fueling Midday," a chapter dedicated to transforming the mundane lunch break into a colorful explosion of tastes and nutrition. Here, colorful salad bowls, hearty wraps, sandwiches, and warm soups await us on our journey. It's about enjoying bursts of delectable energy that sustain you throughout the day, not simply filling up your tank at lunchtime. Come along as we discuss how to make vibrant meals that will satisfy your appetite and boost vitality and well-being in your afternoon. Your favorite part of the day is going to be lunch!

Mediterranean Chickpea Salad Bowl

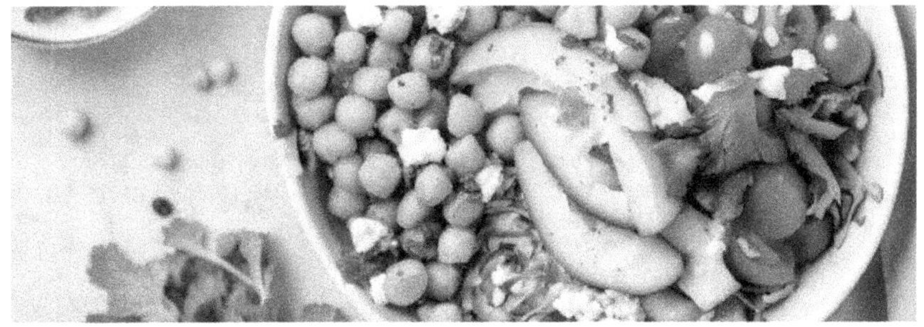

Ingredients:

- Cooked or canned chickpeas
- Diced Feta cheese
- Chopped cucumber
- Chopped Kalamata olives
- Cherry tomatoes, sliced
- Greek dressing

Preparation:

1. Chickpeas, cucumber, cherry tomatoes, crumbled feta, and sliced Kalamata olives should all be combined in a dish.
2. Gently mix and drizzle with Greek dressing.
3. Enjoy and serve right now!

Nutritional Value:

- Chickpeas supply 15% of the daily required amount of protein and fiber.
- Cherry tomatoes include antioxidants and vitamins (20% of the daily intake).
- Feta cheese adds taste and calcium (around 10% of daily value).

Cooking Period: (If using canned chickpeas, add 10 minutes)

Roasted Red Pepper and Lentil Soup

Ingredients:

- Red lentils
- Roasted red peppers (from a jar or freshly roasted)

- Onion, chopped
- Garlic, minced
- Vegetable broth
- Olive oil
- Paprika
- Salt and pepper to taste

Preparation:

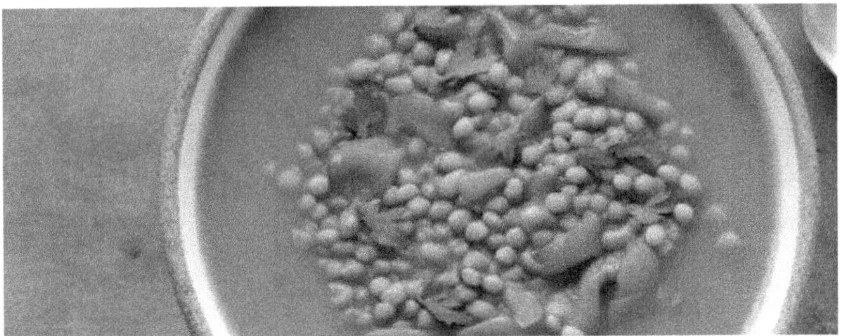

1. Add the minced garlic and chopped onions to a saucepan with olive oil and cook until transparent.
2. Stir in the paprika, roasted red peppers, red lentils, and salt and pepper. Mix everything together.
3. After adding the veggie broth, bring it to a boil. Once the lentils are soft, simmer them.
4. The soup should be smooth after blending.
5. Warm up the dish and add some olive oil on top.

Nutritional Value

- Red lentils supply 20% of the daily required amount of protein and fiber.
- Red peppers that have been roasted include vitamins and antioxidants (15 percent of the daily intake).

Cooking Period: Thirty minutes

Turkey and Cranberry Wrap

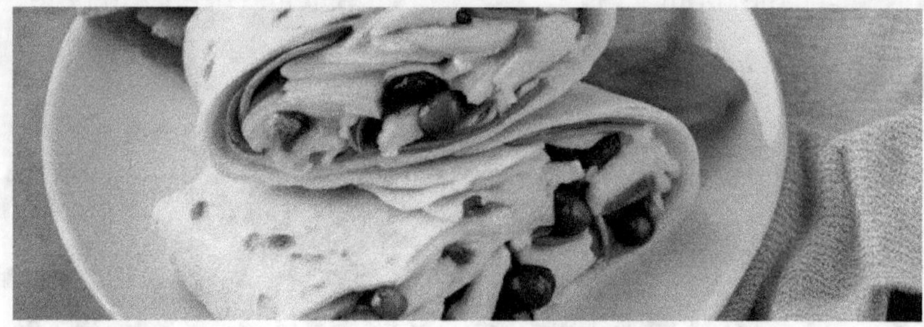

Ingredients:

- Turkey cutlets
- Whole-grain wrap
- Sauce with cranberries
- Spinach leaves
- Cream cheese is optional.

Preparation:

1. Spread cranberry sauce on the whole grain wrapper once it has been laid out.
2. Arrange slices of turkey over the cranberry sauce.
3. A few spinach leaves should be added.
4. Spread a thin layer of cream cheese on top, if desired.
5. After securely rolling the wrap, cut it in half.

Nutritional Value

- Lean protein is found in turkey (20% of daily value).

- Fiber and vital nutrients are provided by whole grain wraps (around 15% of daily intake).

- A pleasant touch and vitamin C (about 10% of the daily dose) are added by cranberry sauce.

Cooking Period: Ten minutes

Grilled Veggie Quinoa Bowl

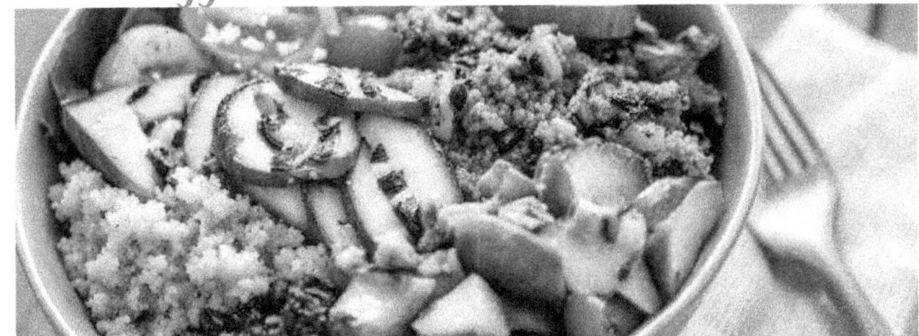

Ingredients:

- Cooked quinoa
- Bell peppers
- Cherry tomatoes
- Red onions
- Zucchini
- Olive oil
- Vinegar with balsamic
- Powdered garlic
- Add pepper and salt.
- Fresh herbs, such as parsley or basil

Preparation:

1. As directed on the package, prepare the quinoa.

2. Sliced bell peppers, red onion, zucchini, and cherry tomatoes that have been cut in half should be combined with olive oil, balsamic vinegar, garlic powder, salt, and pepper.

3. Vegetables should be grilled until soft and browned.

4. Combine quinoa, grilled vegetables, and fresh herbs in bowls.

5. Drizzle with more balsamic vinegar, if desired.

Nutritional Value:

- Protein and fiber (around 20% of the daily value) are provided by quinoa.

- Vegetables that are grilled include antioxidants and vitamins (about 25% of the daily intake).

- 15% of the daily value of good fats comes from olive oil.

Cooking Period: Twenty minutes

Caprese Sandwich with Pesto Mayo

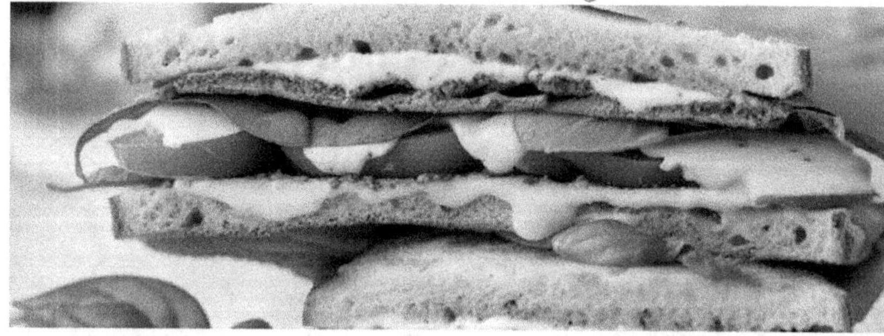

Ingredients:

- Ciabatta bread

- Slabbed fresh mozzarella cheese and sliced tomatoes
- fresh leaves of basil
- Homemade or store-bought pesto mayonnaise

Preparation:

1. Spread the pesto mayo on both slices of ciabatta bread after slicing it.
2. Arrange tomato slices, fresh mozzarella, and fresh basil leaves in layers.
3. Gently push the sandwich closed.

Nutritional Value:

- Protein and calcium are included in fresh mozzarella (15 percent of daily value).
- Tomatoes include antioxidants and vitamins (10% of daily intake).
- Basil enhances taste and provides vital nutrients.

Cooking Period: Ten minutes

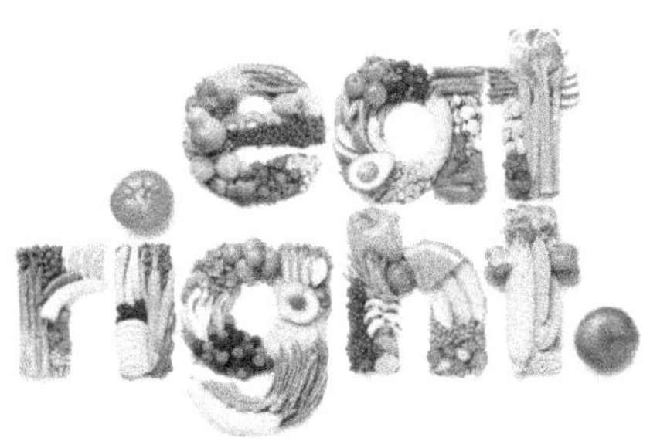

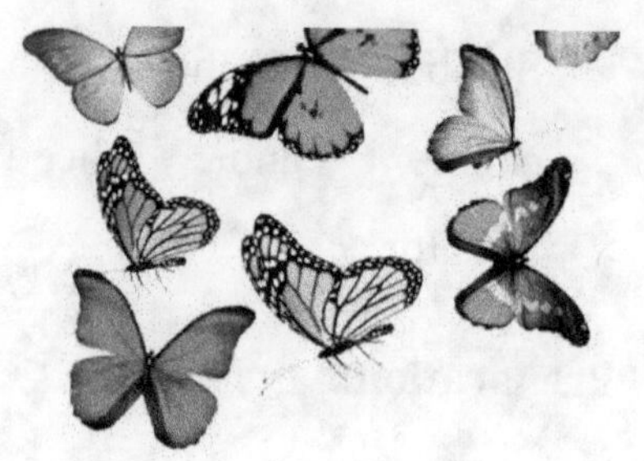

Hey, your ally on this lupus adventure is positivity. When obstacles arise, consider them opportunities for remarkable triumphs. You have a powerful energy in your hope. The better, healthier day after tomorrow? It's not simply a pipe dream; it's a feasible reality. Your upbeat attitude is a game-changer, even if lupus may be unpredictable.

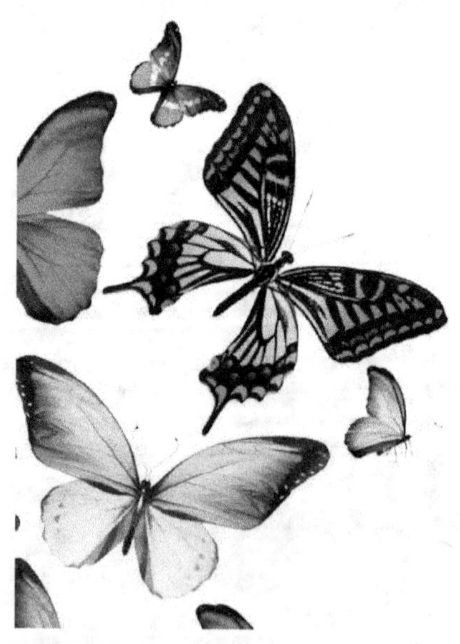

Dinner Delights: Nourishing Your Evening

In this chapter, "Dinner Delights: Nourishing Your Evening," we'll show you how to turn dinner into a rich tapestry of tastes, healthful ingredients, and comforting recipes. Let's look at some meals as the day ends that will fuel your body and please your palate. Every recipe, from delectable grilled dishes to cozy casseroles, is designed to make your dinner table happy. Come share the joy of preparing and enjoying delicious, well-balanced meals and turn every evening into a gourmet feast.

Lemon Herb Baked Chicken

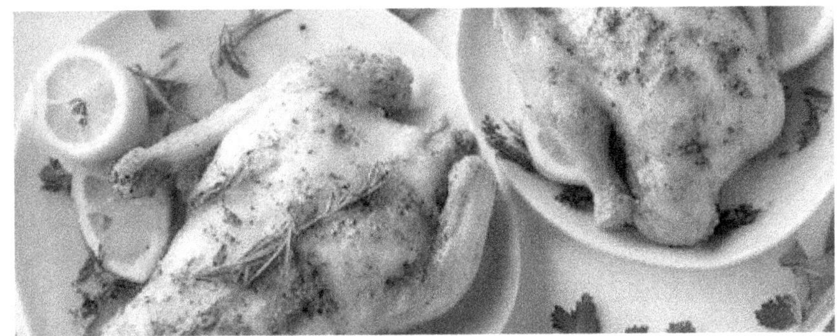

Ingredients:

- Chicken breasts or thighs
- Freshly squeezed lemon juice
- Olive oil
- Minced garlic
- Dried herbs: oregano, thyme, and rosemary
- Add pepper and salt.
- Slices of lemon as a garnish

Preparation:

1. Turn the oven on to 375°F, or 190°C.
2. Combine the lemon juice, olive oil, dried herbs, minced garlic, salt, and pepper in a bowl.
3. Apply the marinade to the chicken.
4. Transfer the chicken to a baking dish and cover the top with any leftover marinade.
5. Bake for 25 to 30 minutes, or until the chicken is cooked through.
6. Before serving, garnish with slices of lemon.

Nutritional Value:

- Protein-rich foods like chicken provide around 25% of the daily required amount.
- 15% of the daily intake of vitamin C and freshness may be obtained from lemon juice.

Cooking Period: Thirty minutes

Sweet Potato and Chickpea Curry

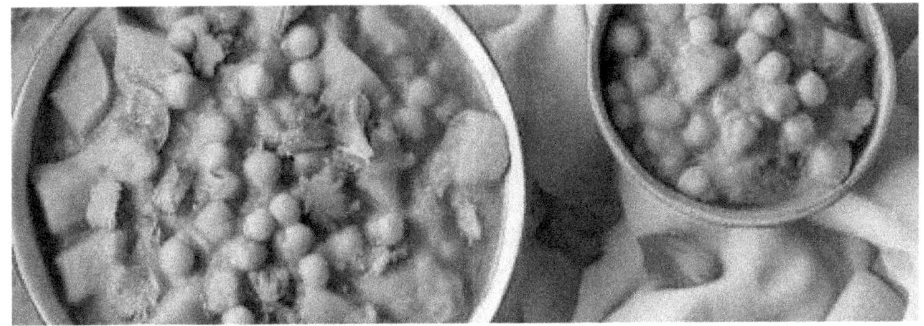

Ingredients:

- Sweet potatoes, chopped
- (Cooked or canned) chickpeas
- Milk from coconuts
- Curry powder or paste
- Chopped onion
- Minced garlic
- Grated olive oil
- Minced ginger.
- To garnish, use fresh cilantro.

Preparation:

1. Add the minced garlic, grated ginger, and chopped onion to a saucepan and sauté them in olive oil.
2. Stir in the curry powder or paste.
3. Add the chickpeas and chopped sweet potatoes.
4. After adding the coconut milk, boil the sweet potatoes until they are soft.
5. Before serving, garnish with fresh cilantro.

Nutritional Value:

- Vitamins and fiber are found in sweet potatoes (around 30% of the daily value).

- Chickpeas provide 20% of the daily required amount of protein and fiber.

- 15% of the daily intake of beneficial fats may be found in coconut milk.

Cooking Period: Twenty-five minutes

One-Pan Garlic Herb Salmon

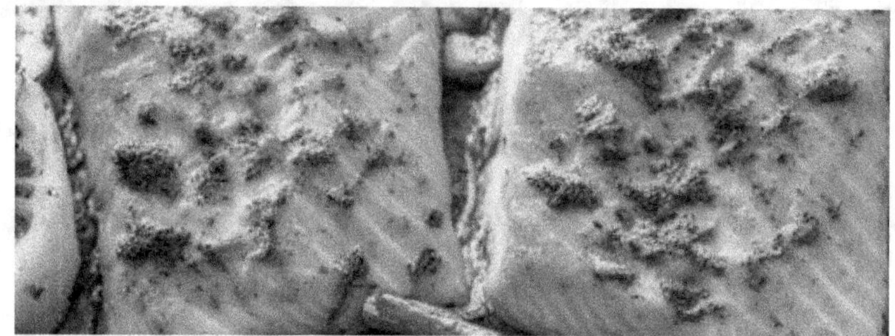

Ingredients:

- Filets of salmon
- Minced garlic
- Fresh herbs (dill, thyme, and rosemary)

- Juice from lemons
- Olive oil
- Add pepper and salt.

Preparation:

1. Set oven temperature to 400°F, or 200°C.
2. Salmon fillets should be put on a baking pan.

3. Add olive oil, lemon juice, minced garlic, fresh herbs, salt, and pepper.

4. Coat the salmon with the combination of herbs.

5. Bake the salmon for 15 to 20 minutes, or until it is well done.

Nutritional Value:

- Protein and omega-3 fatty acids are found in salmon (around 30% of the daily value).

- Herbs and garlic enhance taste but offer little nutritional benefit.

- Vitamin C is found in lemon juice (around 10% of the daily intake).

Cooking Period: Twenty minutes

Quinoa-Stuffed Bell Peppers

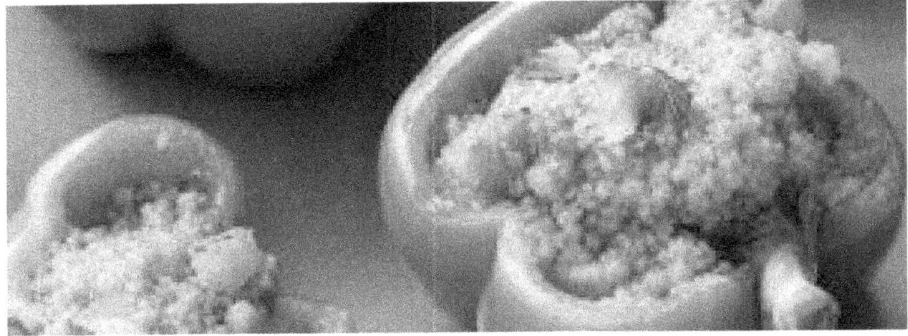

Ingredients:

- Bell peppers
- Cooked quinoa

- Rinse and drain black beans
- Kernels of corn

- Chopped tomatoes
- Diced onion and taco seasoning
- Cheese in shredded form
- To garnish, use fresh cilantro.

Preparation:

1. Turn the oven on to 375°F, or 190°C.
2. Remove the seeds after halves the bell peppers.
3. Combine the cooked quinoa, black beans, corn, chopped onion, tomatoes, and taco seasoning in a bowl.
4. Stuff the quinoa mixture inside bell peppers.
5. Add some shredded cheese on top, then bake for 25 to 30 minutes.
6. Before serving, garnish with fresh cilantro.

Nutritional Value:

- Protein and fiber (around 20% of the daily value) are provided by quinoa.
- Black beans provide 15% of the daily requirement of protein and fiber.
- Tomatoes and bell peppers give antioxidants and vitamins (around 15% of the daily intake).

Cooking Period: Thirty minutes

Bison Burger with Caramelized Onions

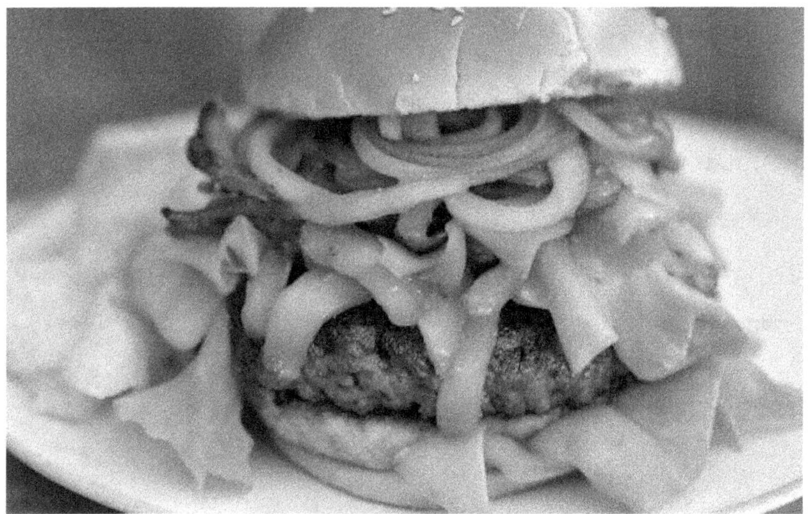

Ingredients:

- Bison on the ground
- Buns for burgers
- Olive oil
- Thinly sliced onions

- Add pepper and salt.
- **Add-ons:** cheese, tomato, and lettuce

Preparation:

1. Patties made of pulverized bison should be formed.
2. Add pepper and salt for seasoning.
3. Thinly slice onions and sauté them in olive oil until they turn brown.
4. Cook or grill bison patties until done to your liking.
5. Burger buns should be toasted before being assembled with optional toppings, caramelized onions, and bison patties.

Nutritional Value:

- Lean and rich in protein, bison makes up around 25% of the daily requirement.

- Onions include antioxidants and vitamins (10% of daily value).

- Cheese is optional but adds taste and calcium (15 percent of daily value).

Cooking Period: Fifteen minutes

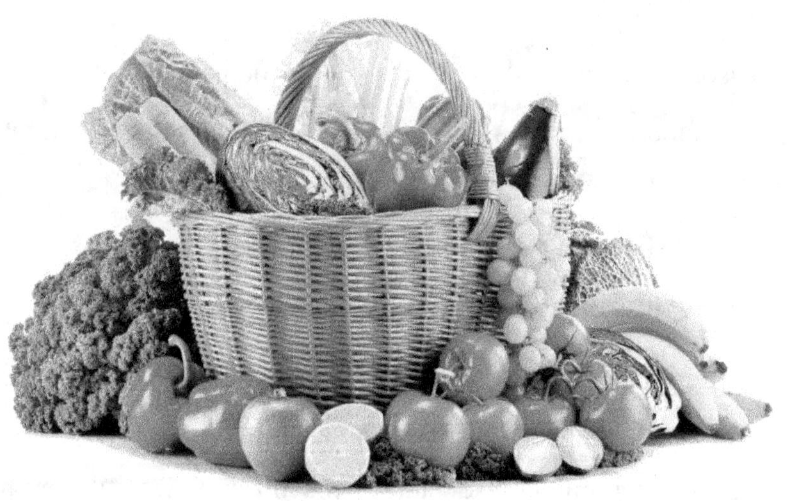

Snacks and Sides for Lupus Warriors

This chapter, "Snacks and Sides for Lupus Warriors," is devoted to creating tasty and nutritious snacks that enhance the experience of those with lupus. Tiny, delicious moments count when it comes to managing lupus. These dishes, which range from filling snacks to delicious sides, are intended to improve the well-being of lupus warriors while fulfilling appetites. Taste with me a variety of tastes that brighten your day, one mouthful at a time. These sides and snacks are more than simply sweets; they celebrate people with lupus who have persevered through hardship and courage.

Trail Mix Energy Bites

Ingredients:

- 1 cup rolled oats

- 1/2 cup nut butter (almond, peanut, etc.)

- 1/3 cup honey or maple syrup
- 1/2 cup trail mix (nuts, seeds, dried fruits, chocolate chips)
- 1/4 cup ground flaxseed
- 1 tsp vanilla extract
- A pinch of salt

Preparation:

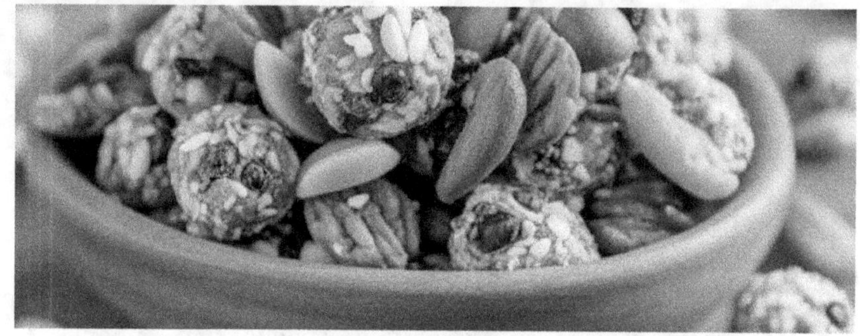

1. All ingredients should be thoroughly mixed in a bowl.
2. The mixture should be chilled for 15 to 30 minutes.
3. Form into bouncy balls.
4. To firm up, refrigerate for a further 15 to 30 minutes.
5. Keep refrigerated.

Value of Nutrition (per serving):

- Approximately 120 calories
- 3g (6% DV) of protein, approximately
- Approximately 2g (8% DV) of fiber
- Approximately 7g (10% DV) of healthy fats

- Added Sugars: around 5
  grams (10% DV)

Cooking Period: All you need to do is chill; no cooking involved.

Fresh Fruit with Greek Yogurt Dip

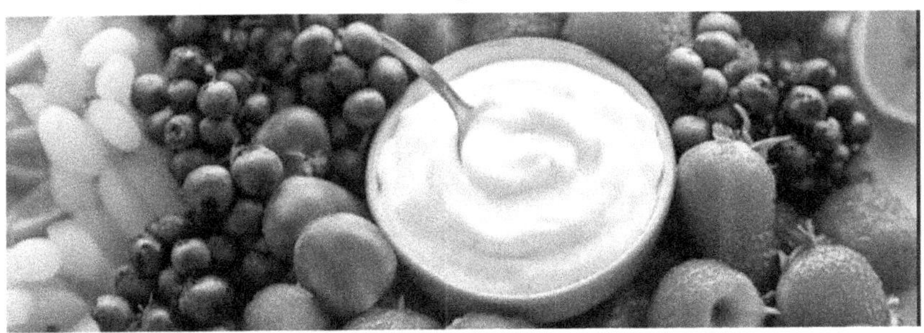

Ingredients:

- A variety of fresh fruits, such as banana pieces, apple slices, and strawberries
- Greek yogurt
- Honey
- Vanilla extract

Preparation:

1. Mix Greek yogurt with a drizzle of honey and a splash of vanilla extract.
2. Stir until well combined.
3. Wash and prepare the fresh fruits.
4. Dip the fruits into the Greek yogurt mixture.
5. Enjoy!

Value of Nutrition (per serving):

- Approximately 120 calories
- Protein: around 8 grams (16% DV)
- Calcium: 15% of DV, about
- Vitamin C: around 20% of the DV
- 3g or so of fiber (12% DV)

Time Spent Preparing: Five minutes

Baked Kale Chips

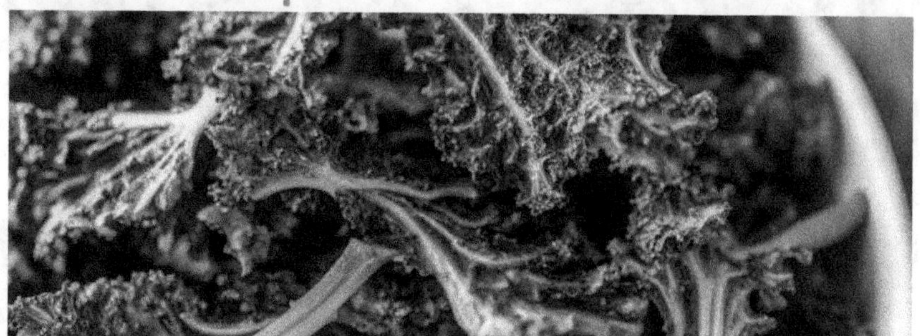

Ingredients:

- Fresh kale leaves, cleaned and dried
- Olive oil
- Salt

Preparation:

1. Preheat the oven to 350°F (175°C).
2. Tear kale leaves into bite-sized pieces, discarding rough stems.
3. Drizzle with olive oil and season with salt. Toss to coat evenly.
4. Arrange kale in a single layer on a baking sheet.
5. Bake for 10-15 minutes, or until crisp, rotating halfway through.

Nutritional Value (per Serving):

- Calories: around 50
- Vitamin A: around 200% DV
- Vitamin K: 600% DV
- Vitamin C: around 50% DV
- Fiber: 3g (12% DV)

Cooking Time: 15 minutes

Herbed Cauliflower Mash

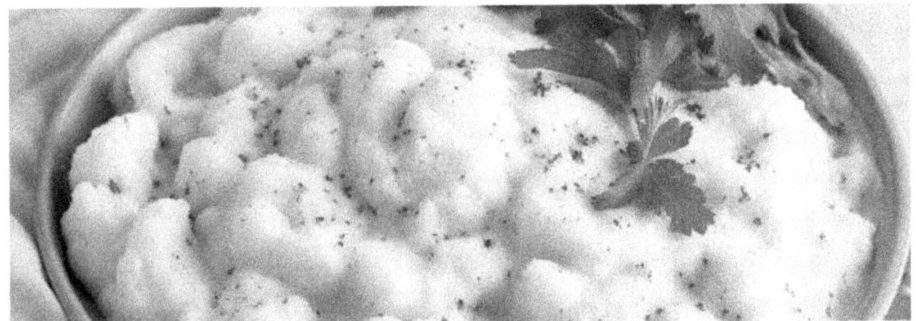

Ingredients:

- Cauliflower florets, chopped
- Olive oil
- Chopped garlic cloves
- Herbs (rosemary and thyme)
- Seasoned with salt & pepper

Preparation:

1. Cauliflower should be steamed or boiled until soft.
2. Sauté minced garlic in olive oil in a skillet until fragrant.
3. Mash the cooked cauliflower in the pan.

4. Add fresh herbs, salt, and pepper to taste.

5. Cook until everything is properly blended.

Per serving nutritional value:

- Approximately 60 calories

- Approximately 70% DV of vitamin C

- Approximately 5g (20% DV) fiber

- Approximately 4g (6% DV) of healthy fats

Time to Cook: fifteen minutes

Guacamole with Veggie Sticks

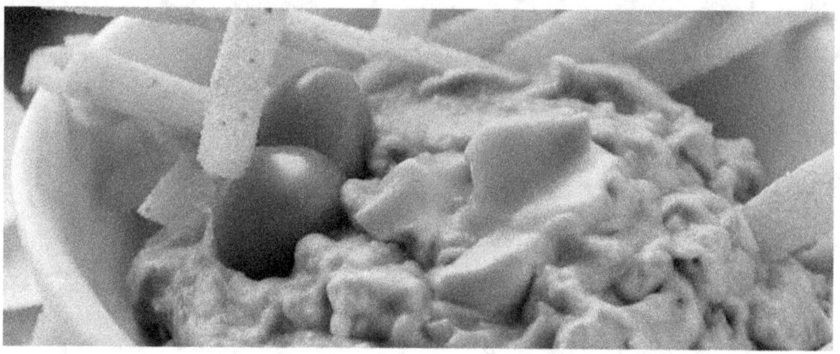

Ingredients:

- 2 ripe avocados

- 1 small red onion, finely diced

- 1-2 tomatoes, diced

- 1 clove garlic, minced

- 1 lime, juiced

- Salt and pepper to taste

- Fresh cilantro, chopped (optional)

Preparation:

1. Cut avocados in half, remove pits, and scoop out the flesh into a bowl.
2. Mash the avocado with a fork or potato masher.
3. Add diced red onion, tomatoes, minced garlic, and lime juice to the mashed avocado.
4. Mix well and season with salt and pepper. Add chopped cilantro if desired.
5. Serve with a variety of veggie sticks such as carrot, cucumber, and bell pepper.

Nutritional Value (per serving):

- Calories: 120
- Total Fat: 10g
  - Saturated Fat: 1.5g
  - Monounsaturated Fat: 6.7g
  - Polyunsaturated Fat: 1.3g
- Cholesterol: 0mg
- Sodium: 10mg
- Total Carbohydrates: 8g
  - Dietary Fiber: 5g
  - Sugars: 1g
- Protein: 2g

Cooking Time: 10 minutes

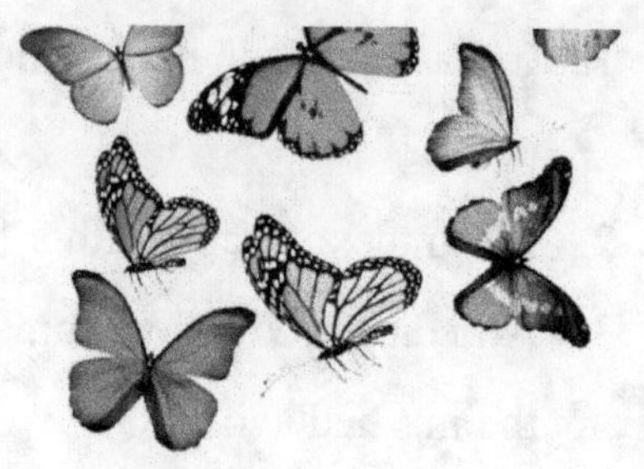

In the battle against lupus, you are not alone yourself. Look around you; a group of fighters is standing next to you. Talk about your victories and setbacks; as we stand together, our power grows. Make connections with others who get the subtleties of this conflict. Your experience is a part of a larger narrative of inspiration, fortitude, and changing the perception of what it means to live with lupus.

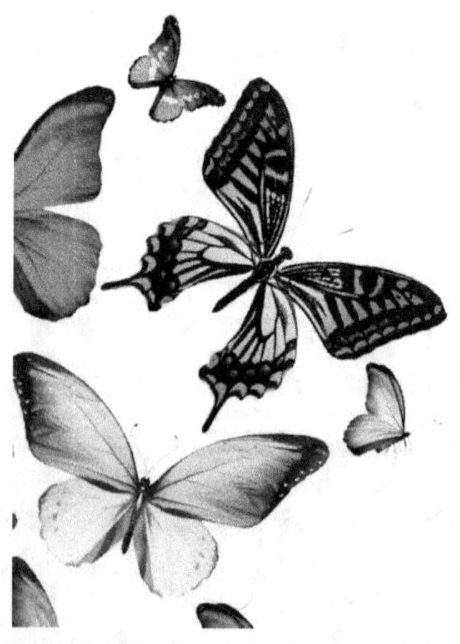

Poultry and Meat Delights

Welcome to "Poultry and Meat Delights," a gourmet journey into the world of savory delight. In this chapter, we'll look at how to create delectable dishes focusing on poultry and beef, with each recipe meant to enrich your eating experience. These dishes, ranging from delicious roasts to tasty grilled treats, demonstrate the diversity and richness that poultry and pork offer to the table. Join me on a culinary adventure where every mouthful celebrates flavor, texture, and the delight a well-prepared meal can provide. Prepare to experience the delectable delights that await you in the world of poultry and meat!

Garlic Rosemary Grilled Chicken

Ingredients:

- Chicken thighs or breasts
- Sliced garlic
- Olive oil, chopped fresh rosemary
- Seasoned with salt & pepper

Preparation:

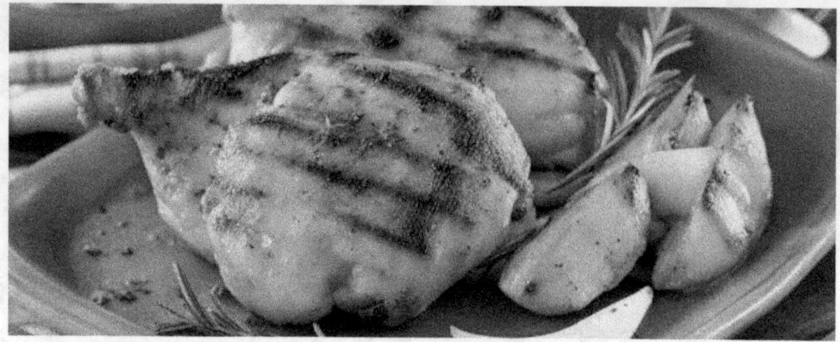

1. To make a marinade, combine minced garlic, chopped rosemary, olive oil, salt, and pepper in a mixing bowl.

2. Marinate the chicken for at least 30 minutes in the marinade.

3. Warm up the grill.

4. Grill the chicken until it is cooked through, about 6-8 minutes each side.

5. Allow it to cool for a few minutes before serving.

Per serving nutritional value:

- Approximately 200 calories
- Approximately 10g (15% DV) of healthy fats
- Protein: Approximately 25g (50% DV)

Time to Cook: 15 minutes (including time for marinating)

Turkey and Quinoa Stuffed Peppers

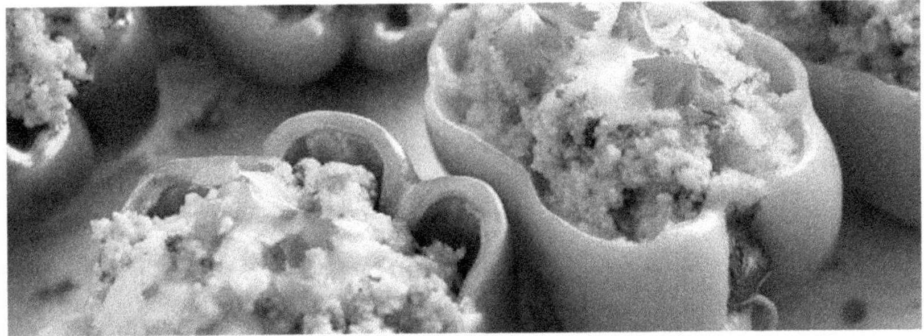

Ingredients:

- Cayenne peppers
- Turkey burgers
- Quinoa, cooked
- Onion diced
- Minced garlic
- Tomato sauce
- Seasoning from Italy
- Salt & pepper
- (Optional) shredded cheese

Preparation:

1. Preheat the oven to 375 degrees Fahrenheit (190 degrees Celsius).
2. Remove the seeds from the bell peppers and cut them in half.
3. Brown the ground turkey in a skillet.
4. Cook until the onion and garlic are softened.
5. Combine cooked quinoa, tomato sauce, Italian seasoning, salt, and pepper in a mixing bowl.
6. Stuff the turkey-quinoa mixture inside the bell peppers.
7. Optional: Shredded cheese on top.
8. Bake for 25-30 minutes, or until the peppers are soft.

Per serving nutritional value:

- Approximately 250 calories
- Protein: approx. 20g (40% DV).
- Approximately 5g (20% DV) fiber
- Vitamin C: 150% of the daily value

Time to Cook: forty minutes

Balsamic Glazed Chicken Skewers

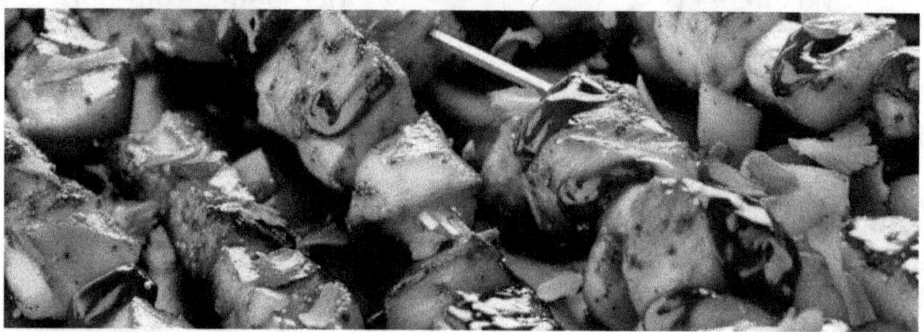

Ingredients:

- Cut chicken breast into cubes
- Balsamic vinegar
- Extra virgin olive oil
- Minced honey garlic
- Seasoned with salt & pepper
- Water-soaked wooden skewers

Preparation:

1. To make the marinade, combine balsamic vinegar, olive oil, honey, minced garlic, salt, and pepper in a mixing bowl.

2. Thread moistened wooden skewers with chicken chunks.

3. Brush the balsamic marinade over the chicken skewers.

4. Grill or bake until the chicken is cooked through, 10-12 minutes.

5. Drizzle with more balsamic glaze before serving if desired.

Per serving nutritional value:

- Approximately 180 calories

- Protein: approx. 25g (50% DV).

- Approximately 8g (12% DV) of healthy fats

Time to Cook: fifteen minutes

Beef and Vegetable Stir-Fry

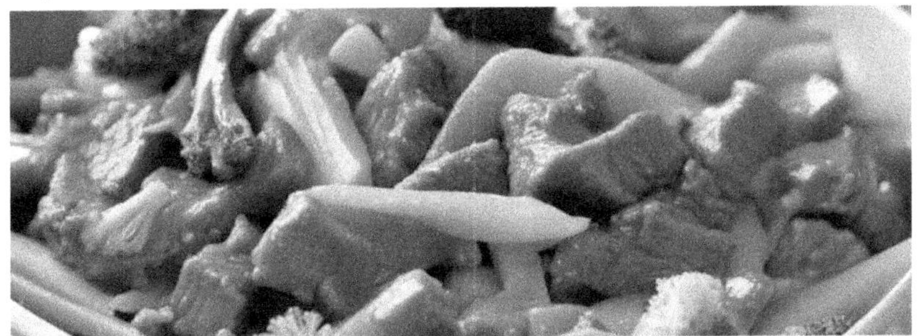

Ingredients:

- Beef slivers

- Vegetable mixture (bell peppers, broccoli, carrots)

- Soy sauce

- Ginger, garlic, minced

- Sesame oil

- Extra virgin olive oil

- (Optional, for serving) rice or noodles

Preparation:

1. Heat olive oil in a wok or pan and sauté minced ginger and garlic.
2. Stir-fry the beef strips until they are browned.
3. Stir in the mixed veggies until they are tender-crisp.
4. Add the soy sauce and sesame oil. Toss until everything is properly blended.
5. If preferred, serve over rice or noodles.

Per serving nutritional value:

- Approximately 300 calories
- Protein: approx. 30g (60% DV).
- Approximately 5g (20% DV) fiber
- Approximately 80% DV for vitamin C

Time to Cook: twenty minutes

Bison Burger with Avocado Mayo

Ingredients:

- Bison ground
- Hamburger buns
- Mayonnaise with Avocado
- seasoned with salt & pepper
- Lettuce, tomato, and onion (assorted toppings)

Preparation:

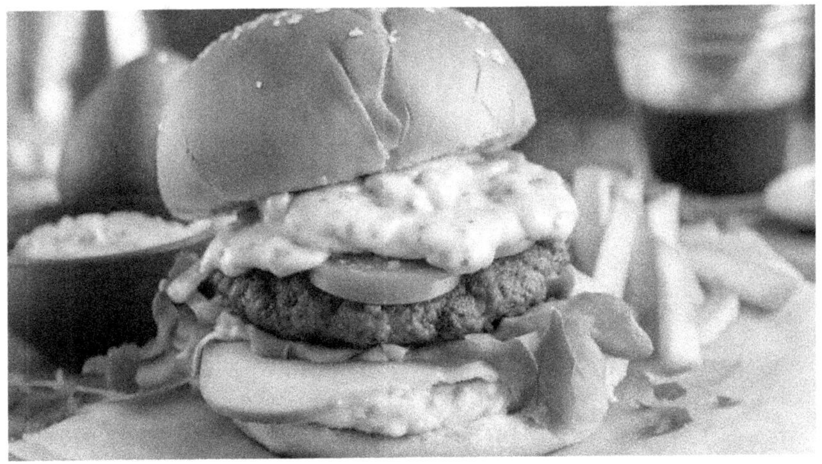

1. Make burger patties out of ground bison.

2. Season with salt and pepper to taste.

3. Grill or cook bison patties until done to preference.

4. To make avocado mayo, mash the avocado and combine it with the mayonnaise.

5. On burger buns, spread avocado mayonnaise.

6. Burgers should be assembled using bison patties and optional toppings.

Per serving nutritional value:

- Approximately 350 calories

- Protein: approx. 25g (50% DV).

- Approximately 15g (23% DV) of healthy fats

Time to Cook: fifteen minutes

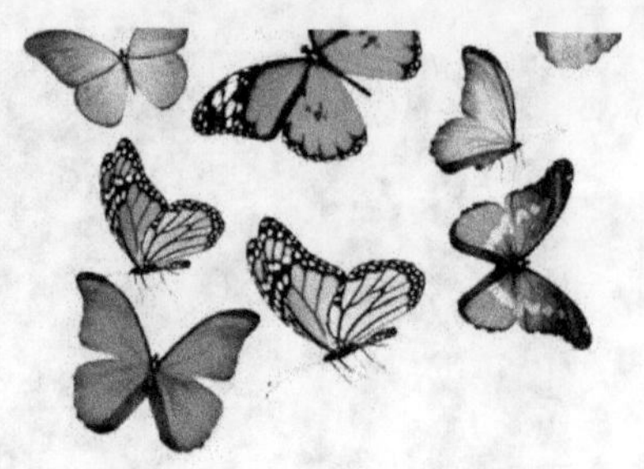

Lupus may throw dark shadows, but guess what? They may be penetrated by your bright light. With the light of your spirit, illuminate the darkness. You can be strong even while you are in agony. Celebrate modest wins and find joy in the midst of difficulties. Lupus does not define you; you are the source of a radiance that may banish any darkness.

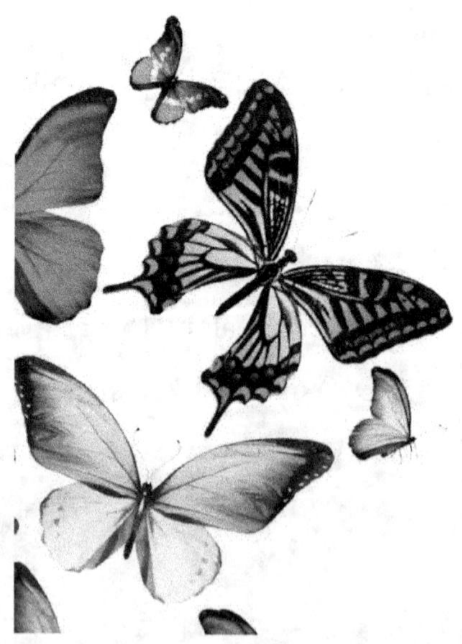

Fish and Seafood Extravaganza

Welcome to the "Fish and Seafood Extravaganza," a gourmet trip that delves into the sea's plethora of riches. This chapter delves into the world of fish and seafood, discovering recipes that highlight the best of the sea. Each dish is designed to capture the spirit of freshness and the sea's delicate tastes, from juicy grilled fish to delectable seafood medleys. Join me on a gastronomic adventure, experiencing fish and shellfish's richness and nutritional advantages on our menus. Prepare for a culinary experience that will take you to the coastlines with every delicious bite.

Lemon Garlic Baked Salmon

Ingredients:

- Fillets of salmon
- Lemon, sliced
- Garlic, minced
- Dill, fresh (optional)
- Olive oil

- Seasoned with salt & pepper

Preparation:

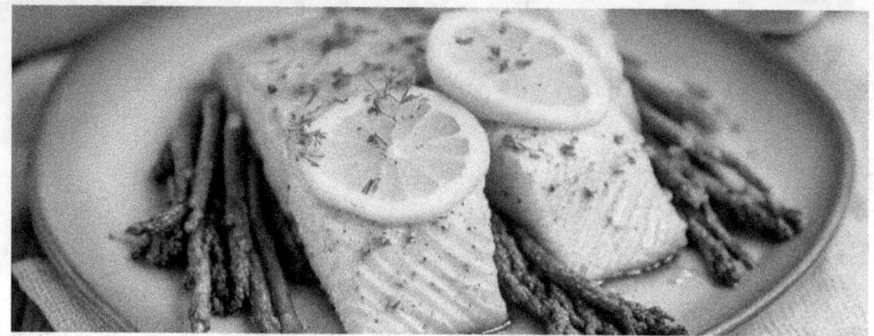

1. Preheat the oven to 375 degrees Fahrenheit (190 degrees Celsius).
2. On a baking sheet, place the salmon fillets.
3. Drizzle with olive oil and season with salt and pepper.
4. If preferred, garnish with lemon slices and fresh dill.
5. Bake for 15-20 minutes, or until the salmon is well cooked.

Per serving nutritional value:

- Calories: approximately 250
- Protein: around 25g (50% DV)
- 1,000mg of omega-3 fatty acids
- Vitamin D: 15% of the daily value

Time to Cook: twenty minutes

Shrimp and Avocado Ceviche

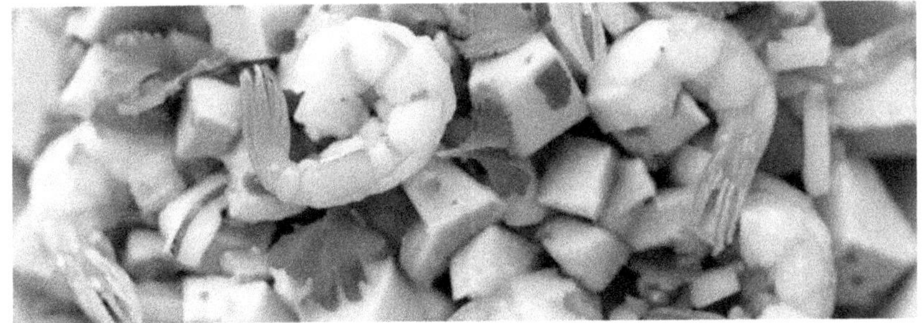

Ingredients:

- Shrimp, cooked and peeled
- Avocado, diced
- Red onion, finely chopped
- Cilantro, chopped
- Lime juice
- Jalapeño, minced
- Salt and pepper

Preparation:

1. Cooked shrimp should be cut into bite-sized pieces.
2. In a mixing bowl, combine shrimp, avocado, red onion, cilantro, Jalapeño, lime juice, salt, and pepper.
3. Refrigerate for at least 30 minutes to allow flavors to combine.
4. Chill before serving.

Per serving nutritional value:

- Approximately 200 calories
- Protein: approx. 15g (30% DV)

- Approximately 10g (15% DV) of healthy fats
- Vitamin C: about 30% of the daily value

Time Required for Preparation: 15 minutes (excluding cooling time)

Grilled Tuna Steaks with Citrus Marinade

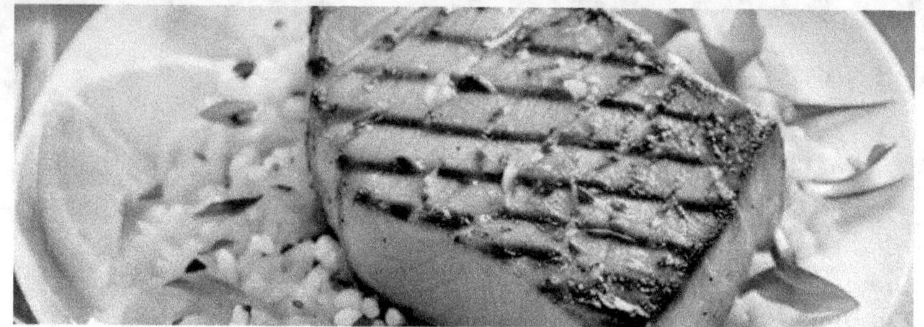

Ingredients:

- Tuna filets
- Oranges Juice
- Juice of lemon
- Soy sauce
- Sliced garlic
- Extra virgin olive oil
- Seasoned with salt & pepper

Preparation:

1. To make the marinade, combine orange juice, lemon juice, soy sauce, minced garlic, olive oil, salt, and pepper in a mixing bowl.
2. Marinate the tuna steaks for at least 30 minutes in the marinade.
3. Warm up the grill.
4. For medium-rare tuna steaks, grill for 2-3 minutes per side.

5. Serve right away.

Per serving nutritional value:

- Approximately 250 calories

- Protein: Approximately 30g (60% DV)

- Approximately 1,500mg Omega-3 Fatty Acids

- Vitamin C: Approximately 20% of the DV

Time to Cook: 10 minutes (not including marinating)

Mango Salsa Tilapia

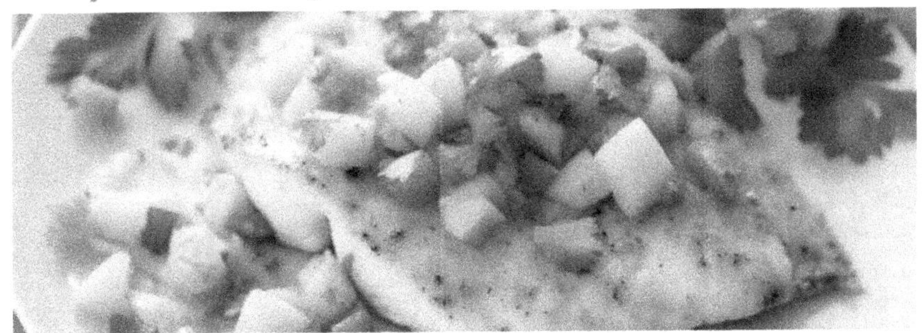

Ingredients:

- Tilapia fillets

- Mango, diced

- Red onion, finely chopped

- Jalapeño, minced

- Cilantro, chopped

- Lime juice

- Salt and pepper

Preparation:

1. Salt and pepper the tilapia fillets.

2. To make the salsa, put chopped mango, red onion, jalapeño, cilantro, and lime juice in a mixing bowl.

3. Cook tilapia fillets on the grill or in the oven until done.

4. Before serving, top the tilapia with mango salsa.

Per serving nutritional value:

- Approximately 200 calories

- Protein: approx. 25g (50% DV).

- Vitamin C: about 30% of the daily value

Time to Cook: fifteen minutes

Coconut Lime Shrimp Stir-Fry

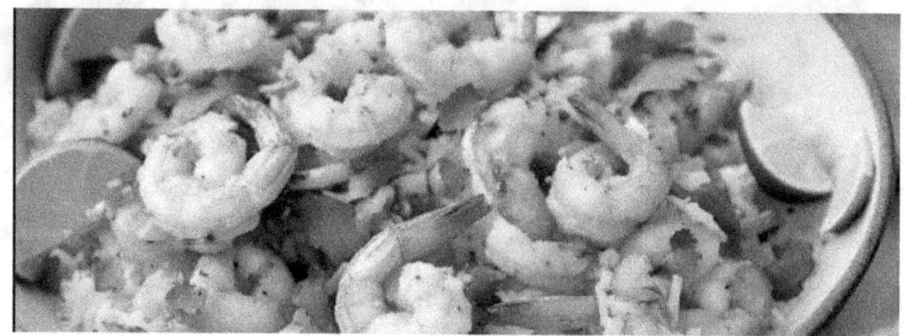

Ingredients:

- Peeled and deveined shrimp

- Coconut cream

- Juice of lime

- Soy sauce

- Sliced garlic

- Vegetables (bell peppers, snow peas, carrots), ginger, grated

- Coconut Oil

- (Optional, for serving) rice or noodles

Preparation:

1. Heat coconut oil in a wok or pan and sauté minced garlic and grated ginger.
2. Stir in the prawns until they are pink.
3. Continue to stir-fry the veggies until they are tender-crisp.
4. Combine the coconut milk, lime juice, and soy sauce in a mixing bowl. Stir until well blended.
5. If preferred, serve over rice or noodles.

Per serving nutritional value:

- Approximately 300 calories
- Approximately 15g (23% DV) of healthy fats
- Protein: approx. 20g (40% DV).

Time to Cook: twenty minutes

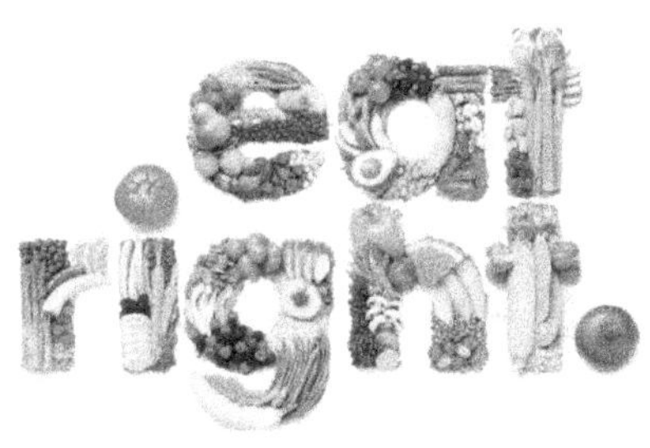

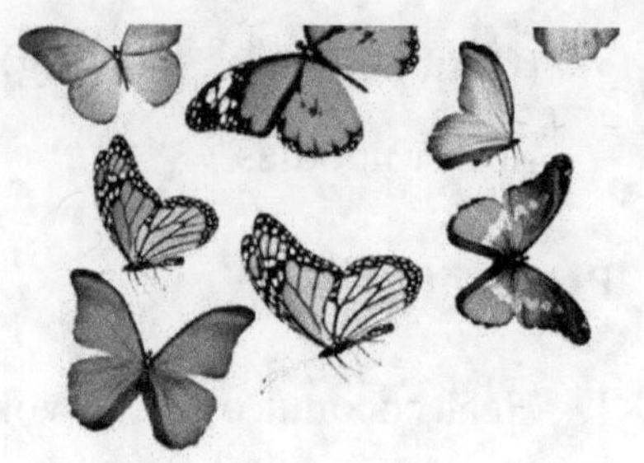

Lupus is not the creator of your tale; you are. Make it into a story of tenacity, success, and unshakable courage. You're not simply a character in a lupus story; you're the one who tells it. Every chapter defies the limitations of lupus, leaving an everlasting stamp on the pages of your extraordinary life.

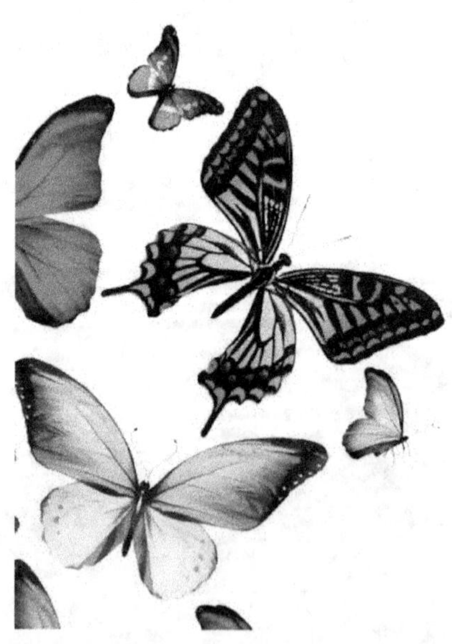

Salads and Soups Recipes

In our "Salads and Soups Recipes" chapter, we welcome you to a world of colorful tastes and healthy delight. We're going on a culinary adventure to learn how to make excellent salads and hearty soups. These dishes, which range from crisp, garden-fresh greens to rich, simmering broths, are intended to delight your taste senses while offering a variety of nutrients. Join me in exploring a variety of recipes that highlight the pure joy of mixing fresh foods in unique and fulfilling ways, whether you want a light, crisp salad or a warm, comforting bowl of soup. Let us enter a world where every spoonful and forkful is a celebration of flavor and health.

Caesar Salad with Grilled Chicken

Ingredients:

- 2 boneless, skinless chicken breasts
- 1 head romaine lettuce, chopped

- 1/2 cup cherry tomatoes, halved
- 1/4 cup Parmesan cheese, shaved
- 1/2 cup croutons
- Caesar dressing (store-bought or homemade)

Preparation:

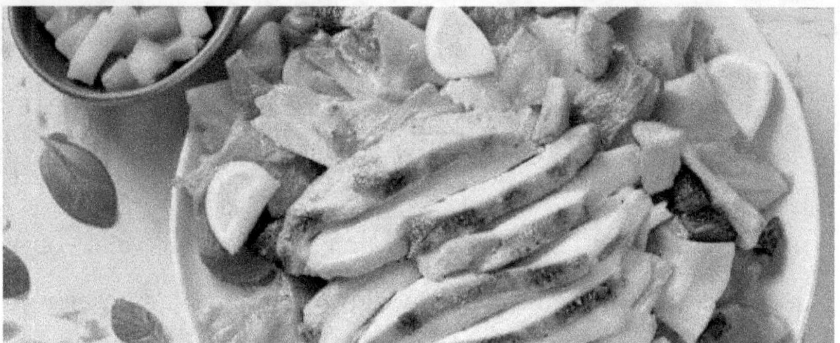

1. Season chicken breasts with salt and pepper. Grill until fully cooked.
2. In a large bowl, combine chopped romaine lettuce, cherry tomatoes, Parmesan cheese, and croutons.
3. Slice grilled chicken and place it on top of the salad. Drizzle with Caesar dressing and toss gently before serving.

Nutritional Value (per serving):

- Calories: Approximately 350
- Protein: Approximately 30g
- Total Fat: Approximately 18g
- o Saturated Fat: Approximately 5g
- o Trans Fat: 0g

- Cholesterol: Approximately 80mg

- Carbohydrates: Approximately 20g

o Dietary Fiber: Approximately 4g

o Sugars: Approximately 3g

- Sodium: Approximately 700mg

Cooking Time: 15-20 minutes

Kale and Berry Salad with Balsamic Vinaigrette

Ingredients:

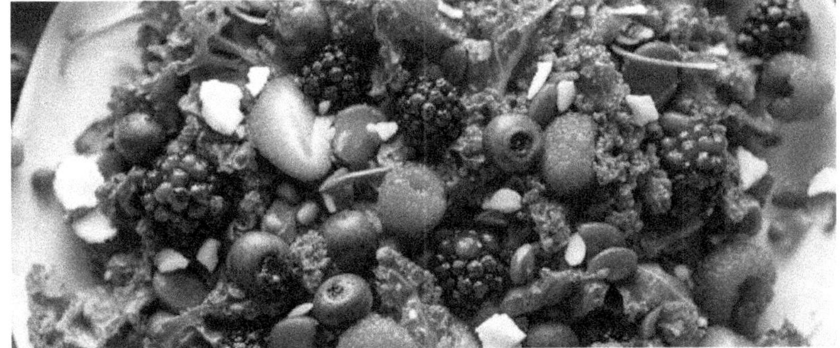

- Kale, chopped
- Mixed berries (strawberries, blueberries, raspberries)

- Feta cheese, crumbled
- Walnuts, chopped

Preparation:

1. To soften, massage chopped kale.

2. Toss kale with berries, feta cheese crumbles, and walnuts.

3. Dress with the balsamic vinaigrette.

4. Toss until everything is properly blended.

5. Serve right away.

Per serving nutritional value:

- Approximately 200 calories

- Approximately 8g (16% DV) protein

- Approximately 6g (24% DV) fiber

- Approximately 15g (23% DV) of healthy fats

- Approximately 50% DV for vitamin C

Time Required for Preparation: ten minutes

Quinoa and Roasted Vegetable Salad

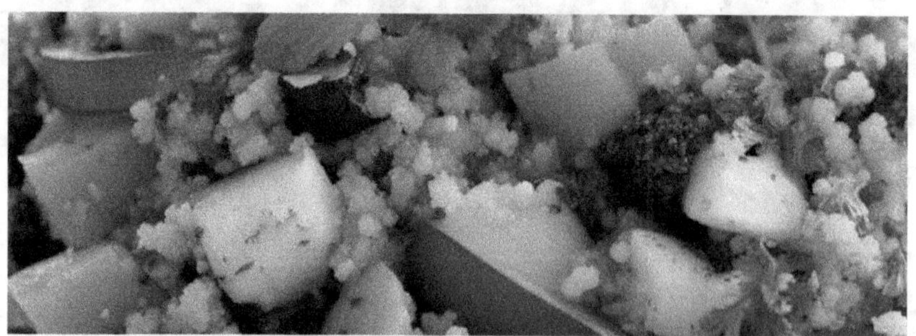

Ingredients:

- Quinoa (cooked)

- Vegetable mixture (bell peppers, zucchini, cherry tomatoes)

- Extra virgin olive oil

- Roasted garlic powder

- Seasoned with salt & pepper

- Fresh parsley, crushed (optional) Feta cheese

Preparation:

1. Toss together the veggies, olive oil, garlic powder, salt, and pepper.
2. Roast the veggies in the oven until they are soft.
3. Combine cooked quinoa and roasted veggies in a mixing bowl.
4. If preferred, garnish with fresh parsley and crumbled feta cheese.
5. At room temperature, serve.

Per serving nutritional value:

- Approximately 300 calories
- Protein: approx. 10g (20% DV).
- Approximately 8g (32% DV) fiber
- Approximately 15g (23% DV) of healthy fats

Time to Cook: 30 minutes (including boiling time for the quinoa)

Tomato Basil Soup

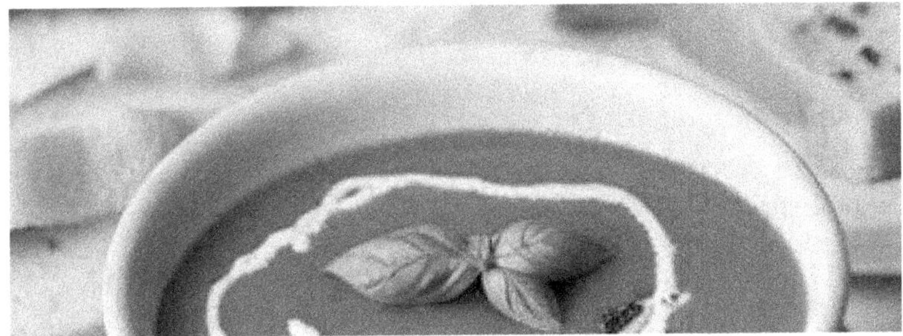

Ingredients:

- Tomatoes
- Diced onion
- Minced garlic
- Vegetable broth
- Basil leaves, fresh
- Extra virgin olive oil
- Salt & pepper
- Optional: Heavy whipping cream or coconut milk

Preparation:

1. Sauté chopped onion and minced garlic in olive oil in a saucepan until softened.
2. Cook until the chopped tomatoes have broken down.
3. Simmer the veggie broth in.
4. Soup should be blended until smooth.
5. Season with salt and pepper and stir in fresh basil leaves.
6. To make it creamier, add a dash of heavy cream or coconut milk.

Per serving nutritional value:

- Approximately 150 calories
- Approximately 20% DV for vitamin A
- Approximately 40% DV for vitamin C
- Approximately 5g (20% DV) fiber

Time to Cook: thirty minutes

Lentil and Spinach Stew
Ingredients:

- Lentils, rinsed
- Spinach leaves
- Carrots, diced
- Onion, chopped
- Garlic, minced
- Vegetable broth
- Cumin powder
- Paprika
- Olive oil
- Salt and pepper

Preparation:

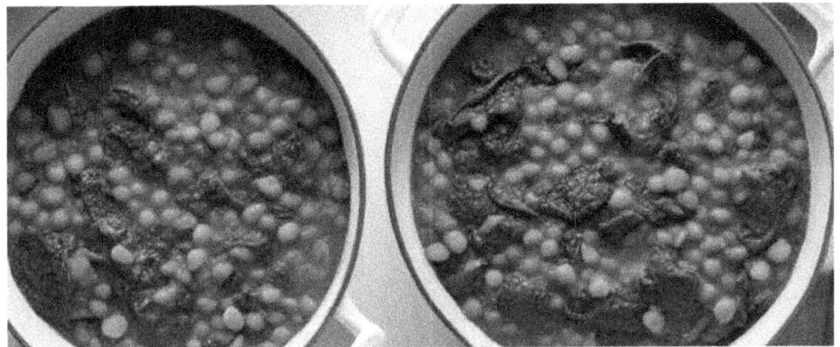

1. In olive oil, sauté chopped onion and minced garlic until aromatic.
2. Cook until the carrots are somewhat softened.
3. Pour in the vegetable broth, then add the lentils, cumin powder, paprika, salt, and pepper to taste.
4. Cook until the lentils are soft.
5. Stir in the spinach leaves until they are wilted.
6. Season to taste and serve.

Per serving nutritional value:

- Approximately 250 calories
- Protein: approx. 15g (30% DV)

- Approximately 12g (48% DV) fiber

- Approximately 20% DV for iron

Time to Cook: 45 minutes

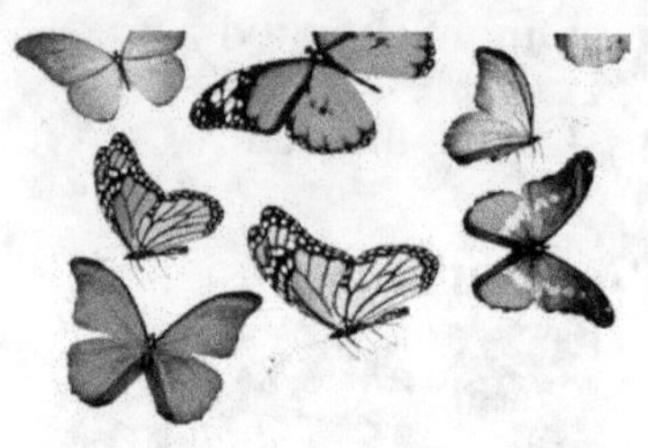

Your journey with lupus is a testament to your incredible perseverance.

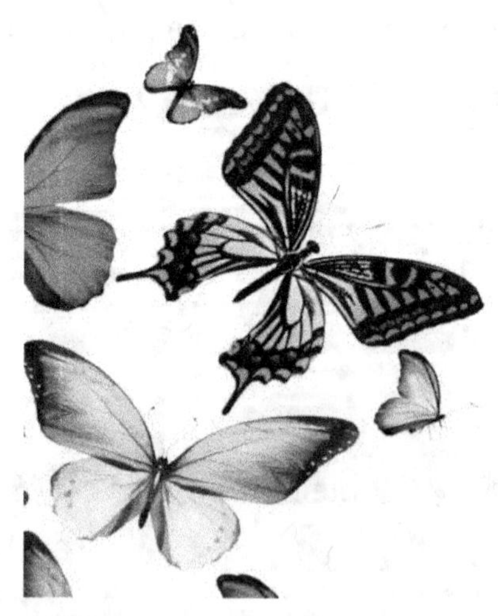

Dressings and Sauces

With these adaptable and delightful dressings and sauces, you may discover the magic of harmonizing textures and flavors, transforming the ordinary into the spectacular. Prepare to discover the key to turning every bite into a symphony of flavor and delight.

Fresh Herb Dressing

Immerse your taste buds in the bright world of our Fresh Herb Dressing, a gourmet alchemy that transforms every dish. This dressing is a symphony of freshness, prepared with a blend of aromatic herbs, including basil, parsley, and dill, dancing in harmony with zesty garlic and brilliant lemon juice overtones. The rich foundation of olive oil creates a velvety texture that adheres to your greens, converting a basic salad into a gourmet masterpiece.

Ingredients:

- Dill, parsley, and fresh basil
- Lemon juice, minced garlic
- Extra virgin olive oil
- Salt & pepper

Preparation:

1. Fresh basil, parsley, and dill should be finely chopped.

2. Combine the herbs and garlic in a mixing dish.

3. Whisk in the olive oil until it emulsifies.

4. Season with salt & pepper and a splash of lemon juice.

5. Adjust the quantities to attain the taste balance you prefer.

Suggestions for Pairing:

- Drizzle over a fresh salad of mixed greens.

- Marinate cooked chicken or shellfish in this sauce.

- With a liberal toss, elevate roasted veggies.

What Makes It Unique:

With the antioxidants and minerals found in fresh herbs, this Fresh Herb Dressing offers a burst of herbal freshness to your foods and adds a nutritious touch. With each pour, it's a flexible companion that inspires you to experiment and create culinary pleasures. Make each mouthful an unforgettable experience by infusing your meals with the essence of garden-fresh sweetness.

Tahini and Lemon Drizzle

With our Tahini & Lemon Drizzle, you can embark on a trip of robust and zesty tastes. It's a versatile dressing that lends a Middle Eastern character to your foods. Tahini, a creamy sesame seed paste, lies at the core of this dish, lending a nutty richness. The vivid lemon juice adds a tart touch, producing the ideal balance. With its silky texture and tempting flavor, this drizzle is a culinary magician, converting the ordinary into the spectacular.

Ingredients:

- Tahini sauce
- Juice of lemon
- Garlic, olive oil, minced
- Salt & pepper

Preparation:

1. Tahini paste and olive oil should be combined until smooth.

2. Continue whisking in the minced garlic.

3. Incorporate fresh lemon juice gradually.

4. Season with salt and pepper as desired.

Suggestions for Pairing:

- Drizzle over roasted veggies for a nutty, citrusy flavor boost.

- Serve with falafel or grilled meats as a dipping sauce.

- To make a tasty side dish, toss with cooked quinoa or couscous.

What Makes It Unique:

The Lemon and Tahini Drizzle combines the silky richness of tahini with the brightness of lemon to create a vibrant and one-of-a-kind taste character. It's an excellent addition to your culinary palette, adding a Mediterranean flavor and a layer of depth to your dishes. Allow this drizzle to be your cooking partner, transforming everyday meals into remarkable culinary adventures.

Tomato Basil Marinara

Tomato Basil Marinara, a delicious and flavorful sauce that encapsulates the spirit of Italian culinary history, is a timeless favorite. This marinara is a symphony of rich flavors, made with large, sun-ripened tomatoes and fragrant basil. Slow-cooked to perfection, it develops a harmonic balance that elevates everyday pasta dishes, pizzas, and other foods into spectacular gourmet experiences.

Ingredients:

- Ripe tomatoes, crushed
- Garlic, minced
- Fresh basil, chopped

- Olive oil
- Onion, finely diced
- Tomato paste

- Salt and pepper
- Sugar (optional)

Preparation:

1. In olive oil, soften finely chopped onions and minced garlic.

2. Stir in the crushed tomatoes and tomato paste.

3. Enable the sauce to simmer over low heat to enable flavors to blend.

4. Season with salt and pepper and stir in fresh basil.

5. To neutralize the acidity, add a sprinkle of sugar.

Suggestions for Pairing:

- Toss with al dente spaghetti for a traditional spaghetti experience.

- Spread as a delicious foundation on pizza dough.

- Serve with fresh bread or mozzarella sticks as a dipping sauce.

What Makes It Unique:

The warmth and richness of classic Italian cuisine are embodied in the Tomato Basil Marinara. Its simplicity emphasizes the freshness of the ingredients, enabling you to taste the pure essence of tomatoes and basil. Enhance your dishes with this adaptable marinara, which will bring the warmth of Italy to your table.

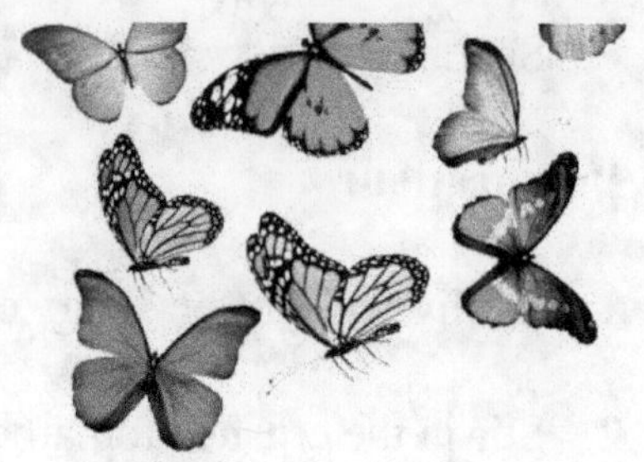

Consider each day to be a blank canvas awaiting your triumph against lupus. Fill it with vivid hues of positivism, drive, and self-love. Lupus is only a speck on the tapestry of your life. Accept the creative process of overcoming obstacles, viewing each one as a chance to add depth and beauty to your wonderful tale.

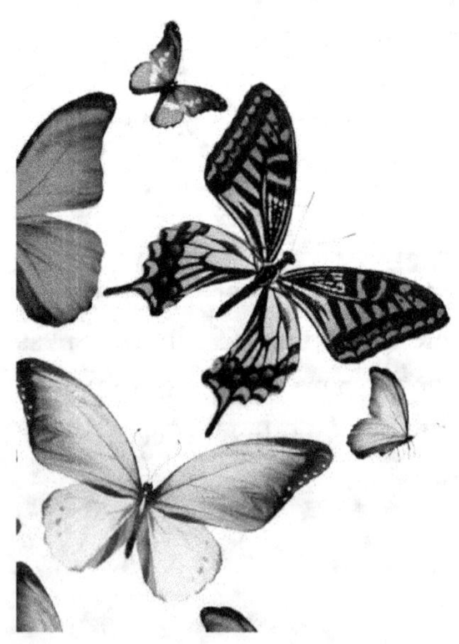

Basics: Lupus Kitchen Essentials

To enhance overall well-being, navigating the kitchen with Lupus necessitates carefully selecting products and utensils. Here's an in-depth look at the Lupus Kitchen Essentials, providing a foundation that promotes health, flavor, and simplicity.

1. Anti-Inflammatory Essentials:

- To benefit from the anti-inflammatory qualities of turmeric, ginger, garlic, and fatty fish (high in omega-3), include them in your diet.
- Whole grains like quinoa and brown rice are high in fiber and important minerals.

2. Immunity-Boosting Fresh Produce:

- Stock up on colorful fruits and vegetables, especially berries, leafy greens, and citrus fruits, which are highly antioxidants.

- Consume cruciferous vegetables such as broccoli and cauliflower, which have immune-boosting characteristics.

3. **Lean Proteins:**

- Choose lean protein sources such as chicken, fish, lentils, and tofu to maintain muscular health.

- To reduce your exposure to additives, prioritize organic and grass-fed products.

4. **Intelligent Carbohydrates:**

- Include complex carbs such as sweet potatoes and whole grains to help with prolonged energy release.

- Reduce your intake of processed sugars and replace them with natural sweeteners such as honey or maple syrup in moderation.

5. **Good Fats:**

- Include healthy fat sources like avocados, olive oil, and almonds to promote heart health.

- Omega-3 fatty acids in fatty fish and flaxseeds are essential for inflammation management.

6. **Kitchen Tools to Make Life Easier:**

- Invest in good knives and equipment for easy meal preparation.

- Consider using a slow cooker or an Instant Pot for easy and time-saving cooking.

7. **Herbs that are good for Lupus:**

- Add lupus-friendly herbs like turmeric, ginger, and cinnamon to your spice cabinet for taste and possible health benefits.

8. **Hydration is Essential:**

- Keep hydrated with water, herbal teas, and infused water with citrus or cucumber slices.

- Caffeine and alcohol should be avoided since they may aggravate lupus symptoms.

9. **Mindful Preparation:**

- Plan your meals ahead of time to save stress on hectic days.

- Portion control can help you regulate energy levels and improve overall health.

10. **Helpful Cookware:**

- To reduce the need for more oil, choose nonstick cookware.

- To prevent potential exposure to dangerous chemicals, choose BPA-free storage containers.

By implementing these Lupus Kitchen Essentials, you may create a supportive atmosphere that promotes health, simplifies food preparation, and allows you to easily relish tasty and nutritional meals.

Lupus-Friendly Grains

Individuals with Lupus must choose the proper grains since some grains might add to inflammation. Here are several lupus-friendly grains that are high in nutrients without worsening symptoms:

Quinoa:

- A complete protein source that contains all of the necessary amino acids.
- Fiber, vitamins, and minerals are abundant, boosting intestinal health.

Rice, brown:

- A fiber-rich whole grain with antioxidants and important minerals.
- Helps to maintain heart health and delivers continuous energy release.

Buckwheat:

- Gluten-free and high in rutin, an antioxidant that promotes blood flow.
- It contains vital amino acids and is high in magnesium.

Millet:

- Grain that is gluten-free and has a moderate, nutty taste.
- Antioxidants, magnesium, and fiber are abundant.

Amaranth:

- Protein, fiber, and micronutrients are abundant.
- Contains lysine, an important amino acid that is frequently deficient in cereals.

Brown Rice:

- Brown rice is higher in protein and lower in carbohydrates than white rice.
- Fiber, antioxidants, and vital minerals are abundant.

Gluten-free oats:

- Gluten-free oats are high in soluble fiber.
- Supports heart health and aids with blood sugar regulation.

Sorghum:

- Naturally gluten-free and flavorless.
- Antioxidant-rich and fiber-rich.

Corn Grits (Polenta):

- Ground corn provides a gluten-free alternative.
- It's versatile and may be served salty or sweet.

Teff:

- Grain that is gluten-free and high in iron, calcium, and fiber.
- Provides long-lasting energy and promotes bone health.

Keep variety and moderation in mind when introducing these lupus-friendly grains into your diet. Whole grains not only supply critical nutrients, but they also help the general well-being of people with Lupus. Always speak with a healthcare provider or qualified dietitian to adapt your dietary choices based on your unique health needs.

Essential Herbs and Spices

Herbs and spices add depth and taste to recipes and may also have health advantages. Incorporating these key herbs and spices into meals can improve the taste while delivering anti-inflammatory and antioxidant qualities for people with Lupus:

Turmeric:

- Curcumin, which has anti-inflammatory effects, is present.
- It gives meals a warm, earthy taste.

Ginger:

- Anti-inflammatory and may assist with symptoms such as joint discomfort.
- It has a tangy, somewhat sweet taste.

Garlic:

- It is well-known for its immune-boosting qualities.
- Adds delicious richness to a wide range of foods.

Cinnamon:

- It has anti-inflammatory properties and may assist in blood sugar management.

- Warmth and sweetness are added to both sweet and savory foods.

Basil:

- It's high in antioxidants and has a somewhat spicy taste.
- Excellent with salads, pasta, and sauces.

Oregano:

- Antioxidants are present, and it may have anti-inflammatory properties.
- Perfect for Mediterranean and Italian dishes.

Rosemary:

- It is well-known for its anti-inflammatory and memory-boosting effects.
- Gives roasted meals a piney fragrance.

Thyme:

- It has antioxidant and anti-inflammatory properties.
- It goes well with anything from soups to grilled veggies.

Parsley:

- Vitamins, minerals, and antioxidants abound.
- Enhances the freshness and brightness of foods.

Cumin:

- Anti-inflammatory and digestive properties are possible.
- It provides a toasty, somewhat nutty taste.

Coriander:

- Antioxidants are present, and it may have anti-inflammatory properties.
- The leaves (cilantro) and seeds each have different tastes.

Mint:

- It is well-known for its calming and digesting qualities.
- It adds a cool touch to both sweet and savory meals.

Use these herbs and spices to find flavor combinations that suit your palate. While these additions can make for a tasty and health-promoting culinary experience, always speak with a healthcare practitioner or a qualified dietitian to verify that your dietary choices align with your unique health needs.

Healthy Cooking Oils

Choosing the proper cooking oil is critical for people with Lupus since certain oils have health advantages while others may add to inflammation. Here are some healthy cooking oils with a good combination of vital fatty acids and anti-inflammatory properties:

Extra Virgin Olive Oil:

- Monounsaturated fats promote heart health.

- Antioxidants such as vitamin E and polyphenols are present.

- Perfect for sautéing, roasting, and making salad dressings.

Avocado Oil:

- Monounsaturated fats are abundant, but saturated fats are few.

- It contains oleic acid, which has anti-inflammatory properties.

- Suitable for high-temperature cooking as well as salad dressings.

(In Moderation) Coconut Oil:

- It contains medium-chain triglycerides (MCTs), which may benefit brain function.

- Because of its high saturated fat content, use it in moderation.

- Ideal for cooking and baking on low to medium heat.

Flaxseed Oil:

- Omega-3 fatty acids, which have anti-inflammatory effects, are abundant.

- Best used in cold dishes or as an addition to cooked items.

Grapeseed Oil:

- Polyunsaturated fats and vitamin E are present.

- It has a neutral flavor that suits it for various cooking methods.

Walnuts Oil:

- Omega-3 fatty acid content is high, promoting heart and brain health.
- Use in salad dressings or as a finishing touch on cooked meals.

Sesame Seed Oil:

- It is high in antioxidants and has a characteristic nutty taste.
- To add depth to Asian recipes, use toasted sesame oil.

Sunflower Seed Oil:

- Vitamin E content is high, but saturated fat content is minimal.
- Suitable for a variety of culinary methods such as frying and baking.

Canola Oil:

- High in heart-healthy monounsaturated fats and low in saturated fat.
- Suitable for a wide range of cooking techniques.

Peanuts Oil:

- Because of its high smoke point, it is suited for high-heat cooking.
- It's perfect for stir-frying and deep-frying.

When choosing cooking oils, it is critical to consider individual health demands and dietary preferences. A balanced and health-promoting diet requires moderation and diversity. Always speak with a healthcare provider or qualified dietitian to customize your dietary choices to your unique health needs.

Alternative Sweeteners

Reducing additional sugars is frequently suggested for people with Lupus. Fortunately, sugar substitutes may add sweetness to your treats without creating blood sugar spikes. Here are several lupus-friendly sugar substitutes:

Stevia:

- Stevia rebaudiana leaves are used to make this product.
- It has no calories and does not affect blood sugar levels.
- Available as a liquid, powder, or granule.

Monk Fruit Sweetener:

- Monk fruit, a little green gourd, was used to make this extract.
- Natural sweetness without the calories.
- Available in powder or liquid form.

Erythritol:

- A natural sugar alcohol found in some fruits.
- It is low in calories and does not affect blood sugar.
- Granules or powdered versions are available.

Xylitol:

- Sugar alcohol is present in some fruits and vegetables.

- It is low in calories and has little effect on blood sugar.

- This product is suitable for baking and cooking.

Coconuts Sugar:

- The sap of coconut palm trees is used to make this product.

- It is nutrient-dense and has a lower glycemic index than normal sugar.

- It has a deep, caramel taste.

Nectar of Agave:

- The agave plant's extract.

- Because it is sweeter than sugar, it may be used in lesser amounts.

- The glycemic index is lower.

Sugar Maple Syrup:

- It is derived from maple tree sap.

- Some antioxidants and minerals are present.

- Select pure maple syrup with no additional sweeteners.

Date Paste:

- Made by blending dates with water to create a sweet paste.

- Contains fiber and various nutrients.

- Ideal for adding natural sweetness to recipes

Brown Rice Syrup:

- Fermented from cooked brown rice.

- It has a faint butterscotch taste.

- Because of its higher glycemic index, it should be consumed in moderation.

Molasses:

- A strong-flavored byproduct of sugar manufacturing.

- It contains minerals such as iron and calcium.

- Use in little quantities to add flavor to dishes.

When adding alternative sweeteners, it's critical to consider individual taste preferences and quantity quantities. Experiment with these options to find the ones that are sweet enough for you. Always seek the advice of a healthcare practitioner or a certified dietitian to verify that your dietary choices are appropriate for your specific health requirements.

Appendix

Lupus-Friendly Grocery Shopping List

Fresh Produce:

1. Leafy greens (spinach, kale, arugula)

2. Colorful vegetables (bell peppers, tomatoes, broccoli)

3. Berries (blueberries, strawberries, raspberries)

4. Citrus fruits (oranges, grapefruits, lemons)

5. Avocados

6. Sweet potatoes

7. Cucumbers

8. Carrots

9. Garlic

10. Onions

Lean Proteins:

11. Skinless poultry (chicken, turkey)

12. Fatty fish (salmon, mackerel, trout)

13. Lean cuts of beef or pork

14. Tofu

15. Legumes (lentils, chickpeas, black beans)

Whole Grains:

16. Quinoa

17. Brown rice

18. Buckwheat

19. Millet

20. Wild rice

21. Gluten-free oats

Healthy Fats:

22. Olive oil

23. Avocado oil

24. Coconut oil (in moderation)

25. Nuts (almonds, walnuts)

26. Seeds (flaxseeds, chia seeds)

27. Nut butters (almond butter, peanut butter)

Dairy and Alternatives:

28. Greek yogurt

29. Almond milk or other non-dairy alternatives

30. Feta or goat cheese (in moderation)

Herbs and Spices:

31. Turmeric

32. Ginger

33. Garlic powder

34. Cinnamon

35. Basil

36. Oregano

37. Rosemary

38. Thyme

39. Parsley

40. Cumin

41. Coriander

42. Mint

Alternative Sweeteners:

43. Stevia

44. Monk fruit sweetener

45. Erythritol

46. Xylitol

47. Coconut sugar

48. Agave nectar

49. Maple syrup (100% pure)

50. Date paste

Healthy Cooking Oils:

51. Grapeseed oil

52. Walnut oil

53. Flaxseed oil

54. Sesame oil

55. Sunflower oil

56. Canola oil

57. Peanut oil

Condiments and Sauces:

58. Tomato sauce (low-sugar or homemade)

59. Mustard

60. Low-sodium soy sauce

61. Vinegars (balsamic, apple cider)

62. Salsa (fresh or low-sodium)

Grain-Free Options:

63. Cauliflower rice

64. Zucchini noodles

65. Coconut flour

66. Almond flour

Beverages:

67. Water

68. Herbal teas

69. Green tea

70. Coconut water

Snacks:

71. Fresh fruit

72. Nuts and seeds

73. Trail mix (homemade)

74. Popcorn (plain, air-popped)

Frozen Options:

75. Frozen berries

76. Frozen vegetables (broccoli, spinach)

77. Frozen fish fillets

78. Cauliflower gnocchi (gluten-free)

Extras:

79. Herbed spices for lupus-friendly recipes

80. Lupus-friendly multivitamins or supplements (consult with healthcare provider)

Adapt this grocery shopping list based on personal preferences, dietary needs, and any specific recommendations from healthcare professionals. Prioritize whole, nutrient-dense foods while minimizing processed items to support overall health and lupus management.

7-Day Lupus-Friendly Meal Plan

Day 1:

Breakfast:

- *Tropical Sunrise Smoothie Bowl*

Snack:

- *Trail Mix Energy Bites*

Lunch:

- *Mediterranean Chickpea Salad Bowl*

Snack:

- *Fresh Fruit with Greek Yogurt Dip*

Dinner:

- *Lemon Herb Baked Chicken*

Day 2:

Breakfast:

- *Quinoa and Berry Breakfast Parfait*

Snack:

- *Baked Kale Chips*

Lunch:

- *Roasted Red Pepper and Lentil Soup*

Snack:

- *Guacamole with Veggie Sticks*

Dinner:

- *Sweet Potato and Chickpea Curry*

Day 3:

Breakfast:

- *Spinach and Feta Breakfast Wrap*

Snack:

- *Herbed Cauliflower Mash*

Lunch:

- *Turkey and Cranberry Wrap*

Snack:

- *Fresh Fruit with Greek Yogurt Dip*

Dinner:

- *One-Pan Garlic Herb Salmon*

Day 4:

Breakfast:

- *Blueberry Almond Overnight Oats*

Snack:

- *Trail Mix Energy Bites*

Lunch:

- *Grilled Veggie Quinoa Bowl*

Snack:

- *Herbed Cauliflower Mash*

Dinner:

- *Quinoa-Stuffed Bell Peppers*

Day 5:

Breakfast:

- *Avocado and Smoked Salmon Breakfast Toast*

Snack:

- *Fresh Fruit with Greek Yogurt Dip*

Lunch:

- *Bison Burger with Caramelized Onions*

Snack:

- *Baked Kale Chips*

Dinner:

- *Balsamic Glazed Chicken Skewers*

Day 6:

Breakfast:

- *Mango Salsa Tilapia*

Snack:

- *Guacamole with Veggie Sticks*

Lunch:

- *Coconut Lime Shrimp Stir-Fry*

Snack:

- *Trail Mix Energy Bites*

Dinner:

- *Quinoa and Roasted Vegetable Salad*

Day 7:

Breakfast:

- *Tropical Sunrise Smoothie Bowl*

Snack:

- *Herbed Cauliflower Mash*

Lunch:

- *Lemon Garlic Baked Salmon*

Snack:

- *Fresh Fruit with Greek Yogurt Dip*

Dinner:

- *Lentil and Spinach Stew*

Adjust portion sizes based on individual preferences and dietary needs. Always consult with a healthcare professional or a registered dietitian for personalized advice. Enjoy nourishing, delicious meals to support your well-being on your lupus journey

For further Questions and advice reach out on

joanmilonehelpdesk@gmail.com

Thank You

I'm writing this with a heart full of gratitude for your kind words and the time you took to read my book, knowing that my words have resonated with you is a reward beyond measure. Thank you again for your appreciation and for being a part of this literary journey.

Warmly,

Joan

>>>

30 Days
Meal
Planner

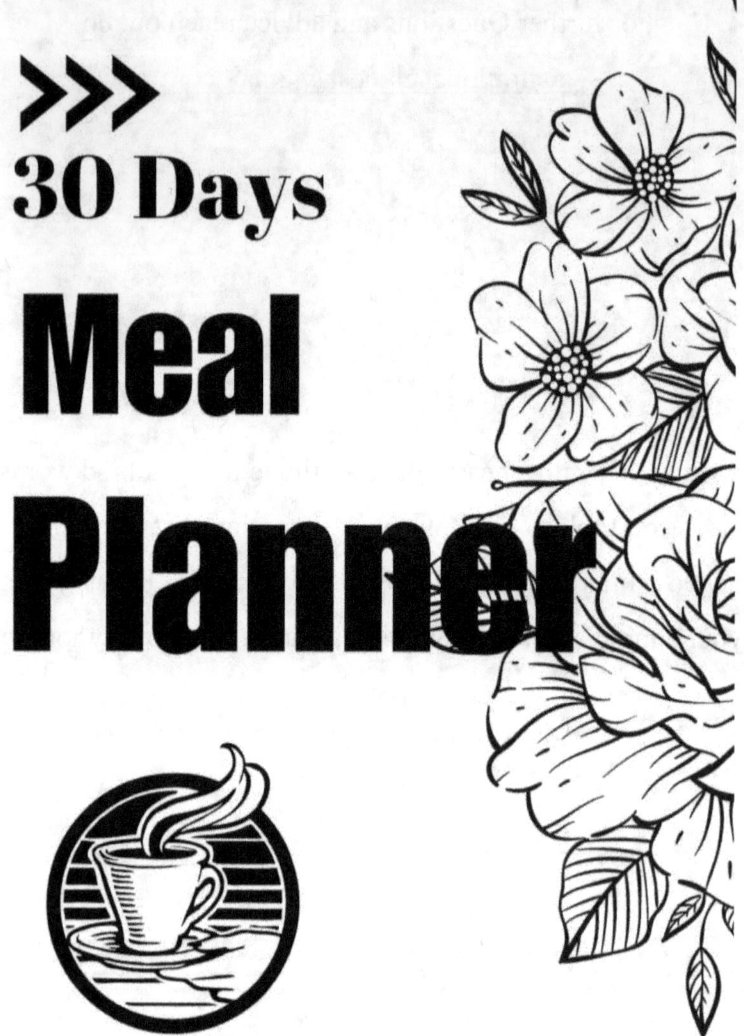

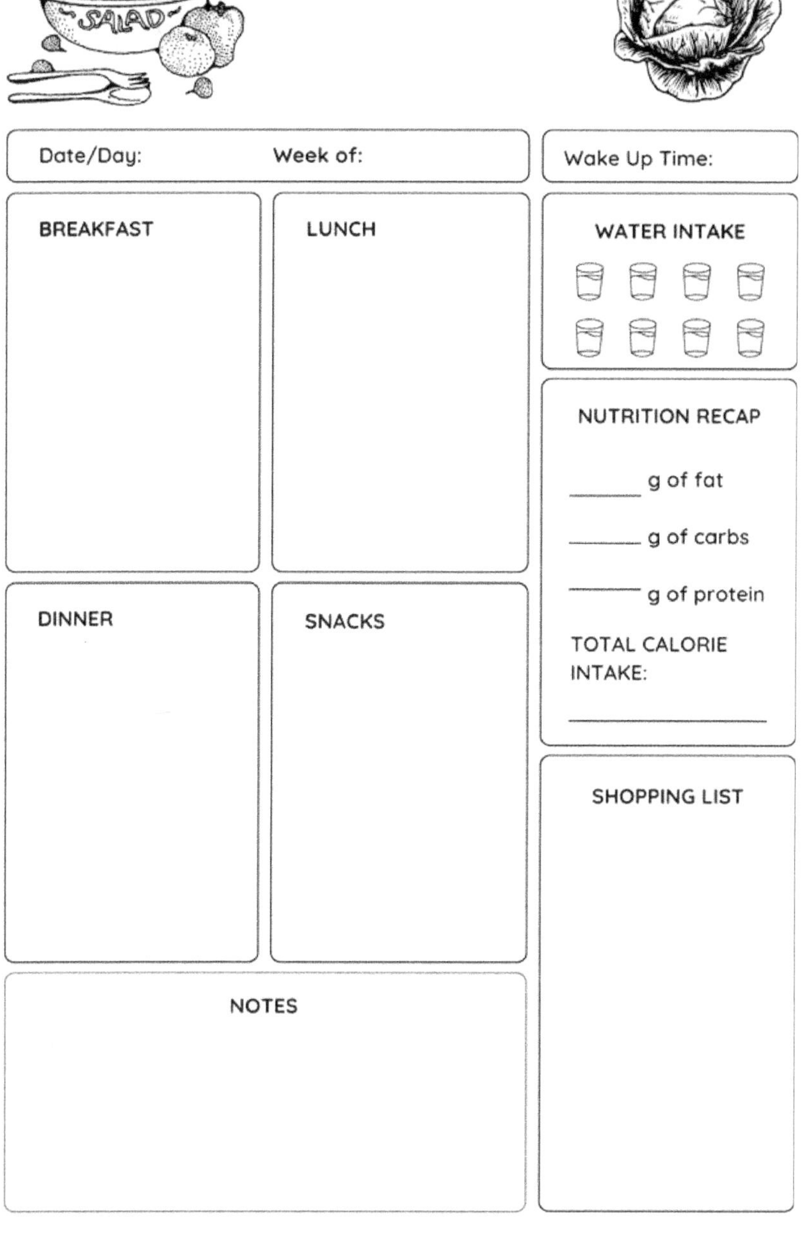
Date/Day:
Week of:
Wake Up Time:
BREAKFAST
LUNCH
WATER INTAKE
NUTRITION RECAP
_______ g of fat
_______ g of carbs
_______ g of protein
TOTAL CALORIE INTAKE:
DINNER
SNACKS
SHOPPING LIST
NOTES

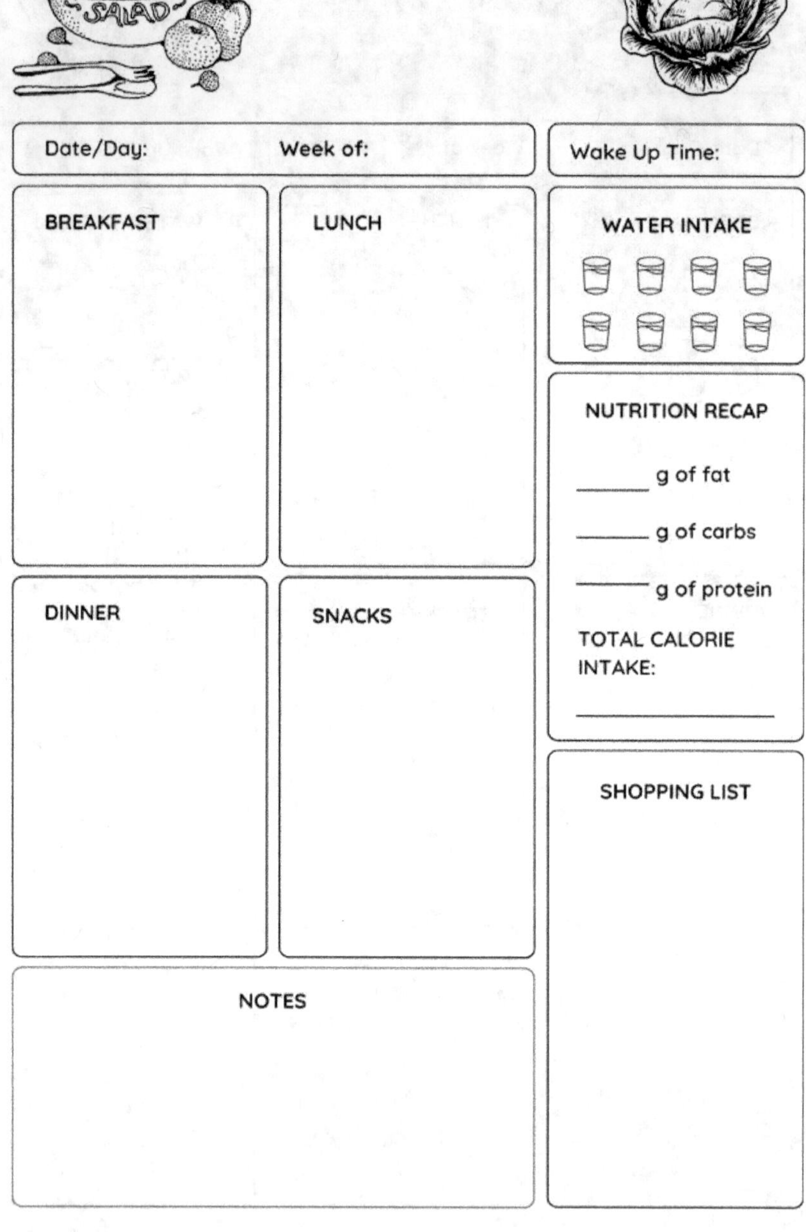

| Date/Day: | Week of: | Wake Up Time: |

BREAKFAST

LUNCH

WATER INTAKE

NUTRITION RECAP

______ g of fat

______ g of carbs

______ g of protein

TOTAL CALORIE INTAKE:

____

DINNER

SNACKS

SHOPPING LIST

NOTES

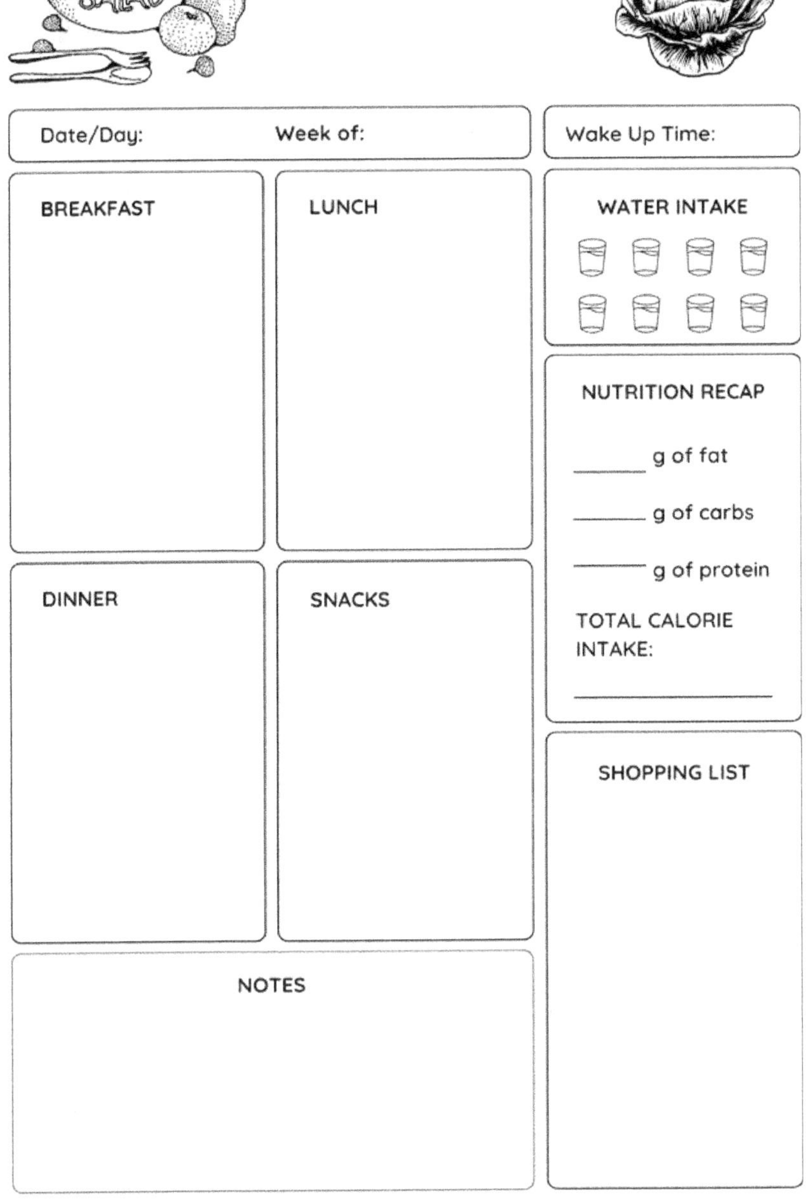

Date/Day:
Week of:
Wake Up Time:
BREAKFAST
LUNCH
WATER INTAKE
NUTRITION RECAP
_______ g of fat
_______ g of carbs
_______ g of protein
TOTAL CALORIE INTAKE:
DINNER
SNACKS
SHOPPING LIST
NOTES

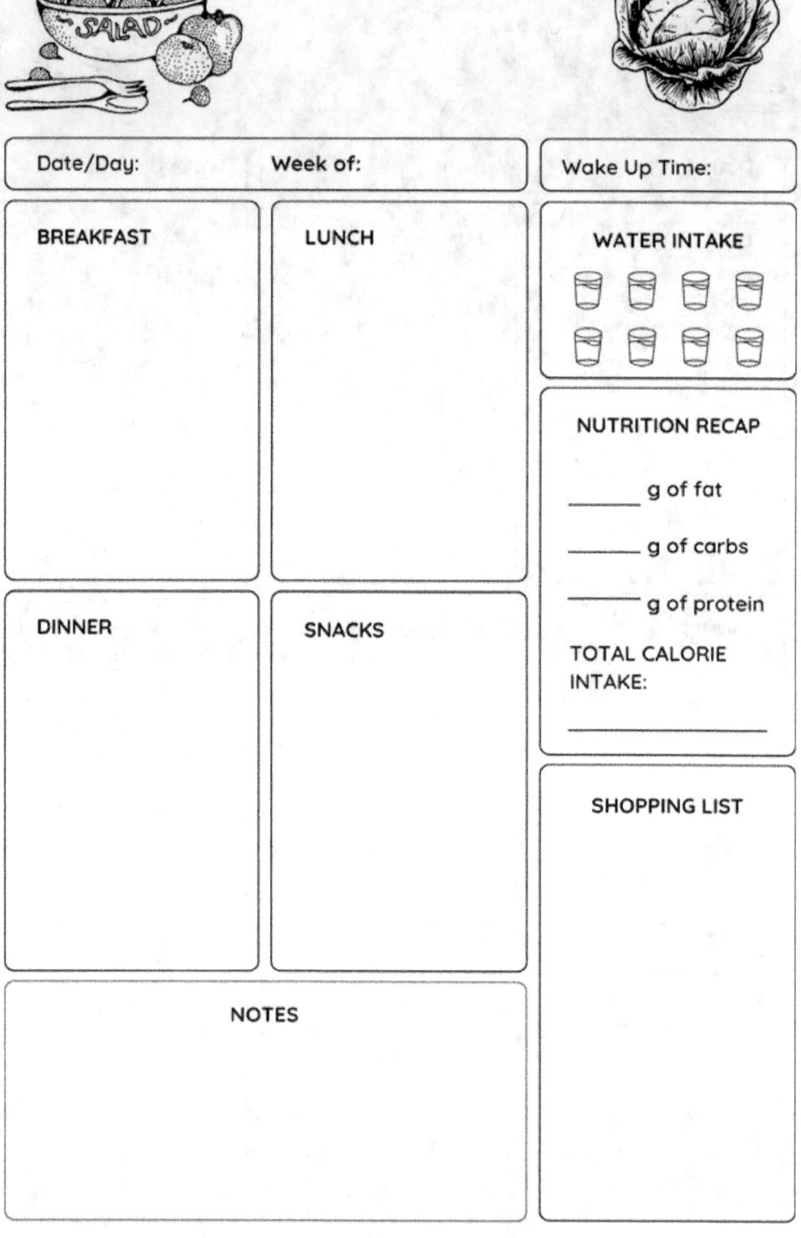

Date/Day: Week of: Wake Up Time:

BREAKFAST

LUNCH

WATER INTAKE

NUTRITION RECAP

_______ g of fat

_______ g of carbs

_______ g of protein

TOTAL CALORIE INTAKE:

DINNER

SNACKS

SHOPPING LIST

NOTES

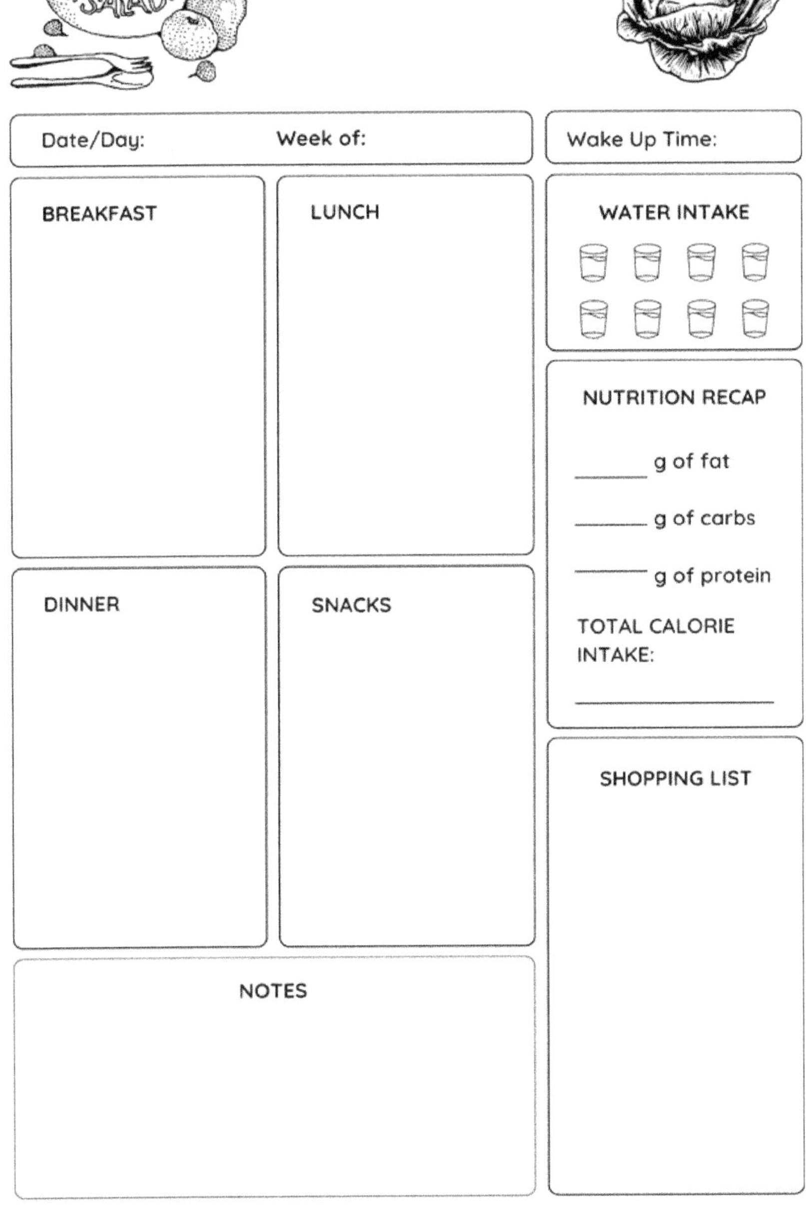

| Date/Day: | Week of: | Wake Up Time: |

BREAKFAST

LUNCH

WATER INTAKE

NUTRITION RECAP

________ g of fat

________ g of carbs

________ g of protein

TOTAL CALORIE INTAKE:

____

DINNER

SNACKS

SHOPPING LIST

NOTES

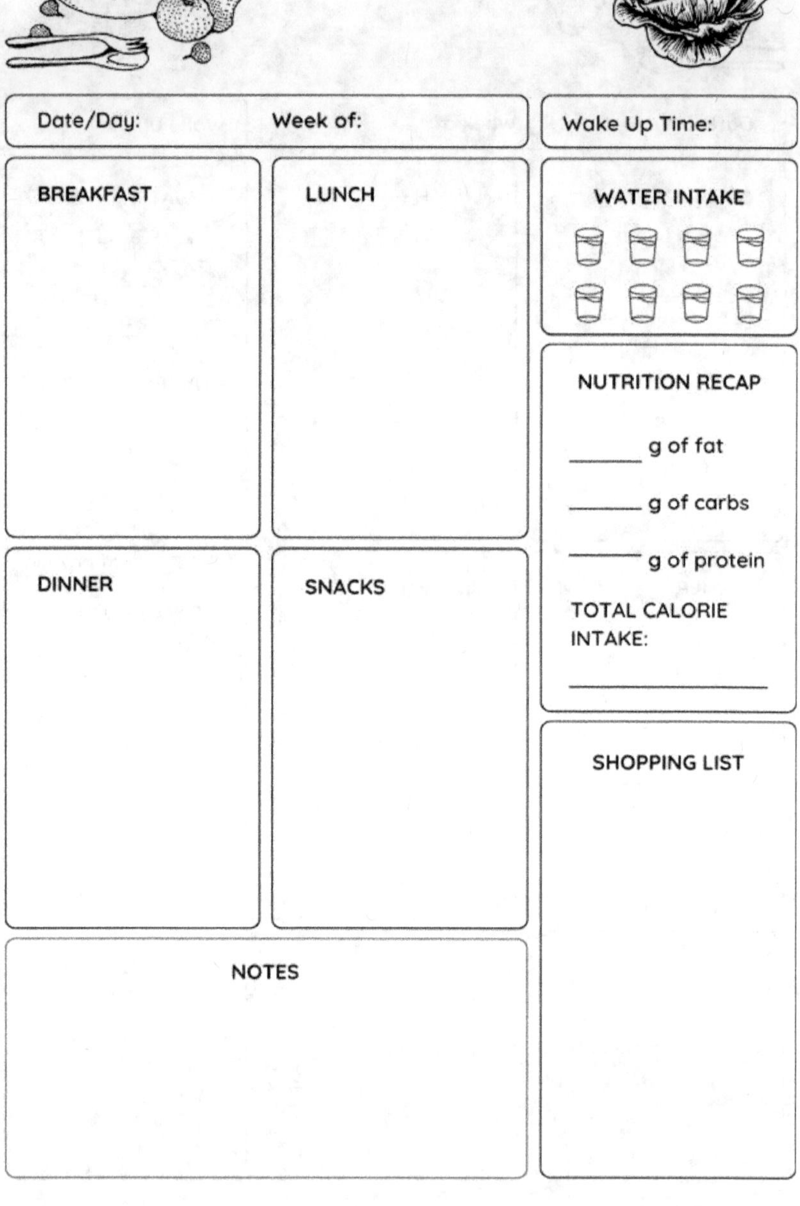

Date/Day: Week of: Wake Up Time:

BREAKFAST

LUNCH

WATER INTAKE

NUTRITION RECAP

_______ g of fat

_______ g of carbs

_______ g of protein

TOTAL CALORIE INTAKE:

DINNER

SNACKS

SHOPPING LIST

NOTES

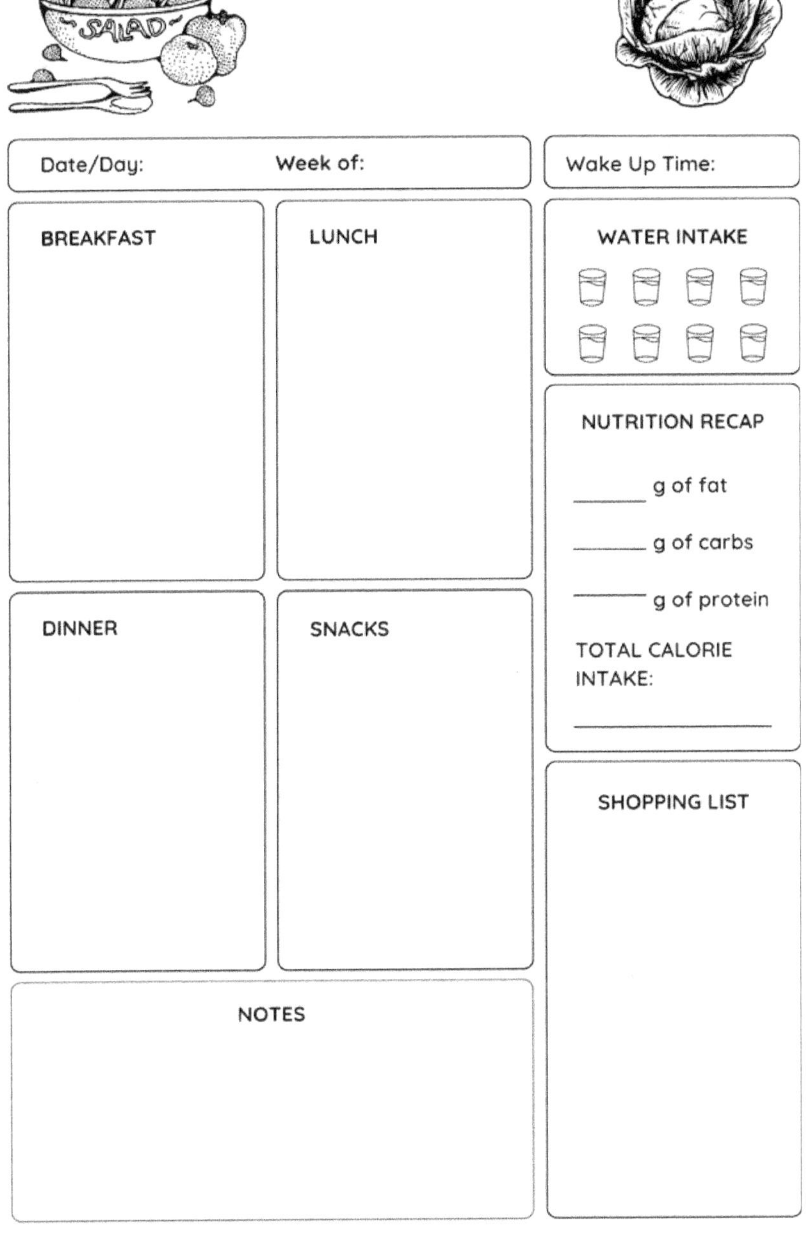

Date/Day: Week of:

Wake Up Time:

BREAKFAST

LUNCH

WATER INTAKE

NUTRITION RECAP

_______ g of fat

_______ g of carbs

_______ g of protein

TOTAL CALORIE INTAKE:

____

DINNER

SNACKS

SHOPPING LIST

NOTES

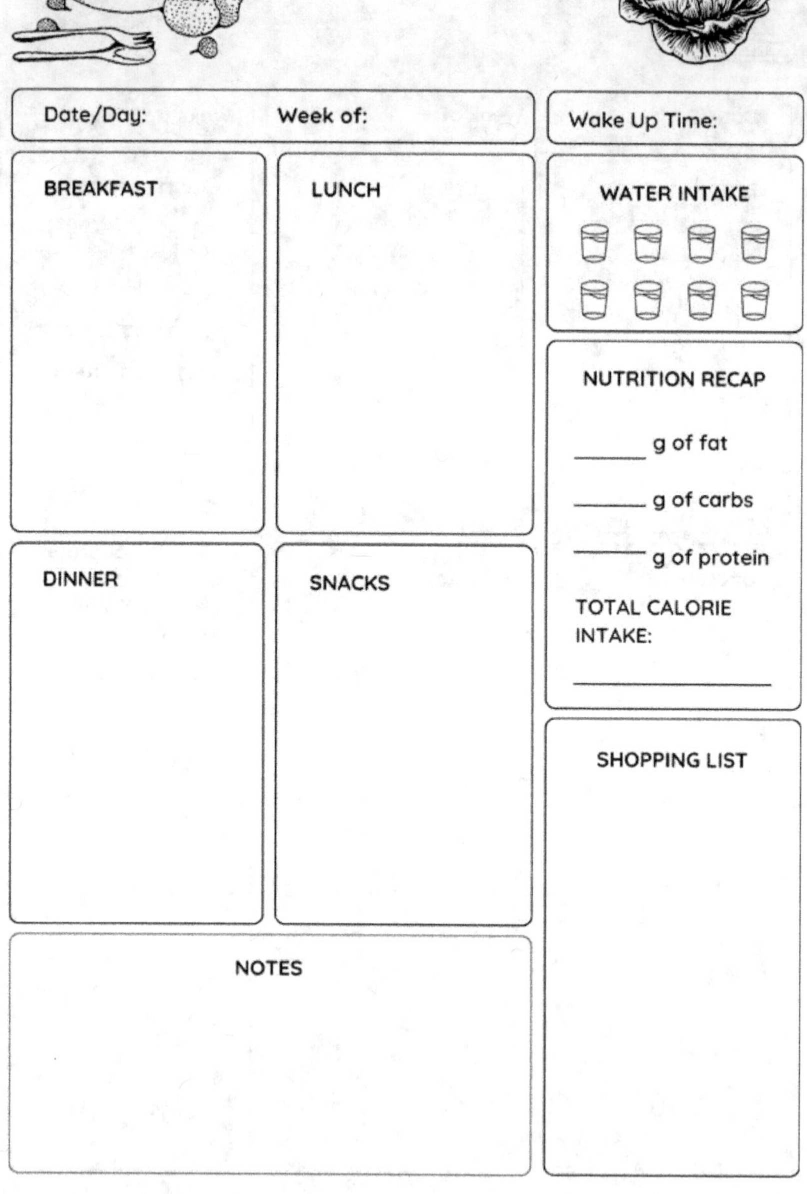

Date/Day: Week of:

Wake Up Time:

BREAKFAST

LUNCH

WATER INTAKE

NUTRITION RECAP

________ g of fat

________ g of carbs

________ g of protein

TOTAL CALORIE INTAKE:

____

DINNER

SNACKS

SHOPPING LIST

NOTES

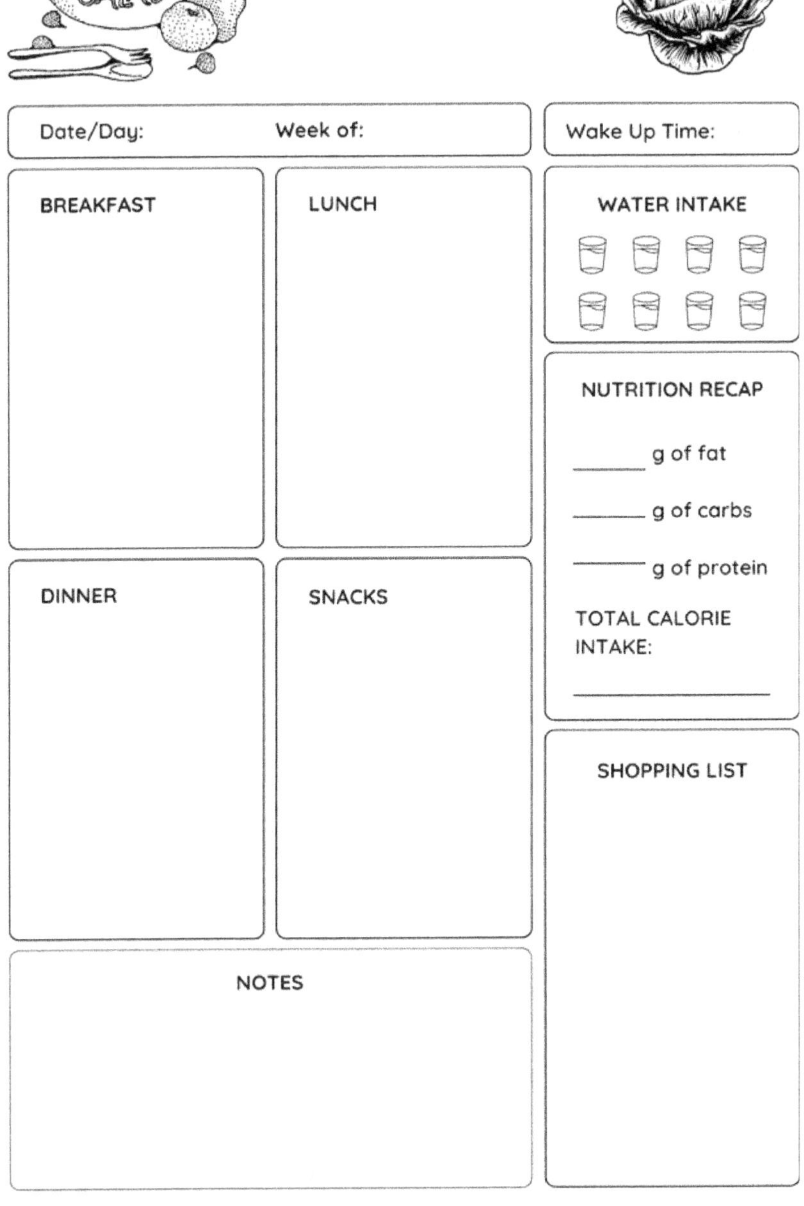

Date/Day:
Week of:
Wake Up Time:
BREAKFAST
LUNCH
WATER INTAKE
NUTRITION RECAP
_______ g of fat
_______ g of carbs
_______ g of protein
TOTAL CALORIE INTAKE:
DINNER
SNACKS
SHOPPING LIST
NOTES

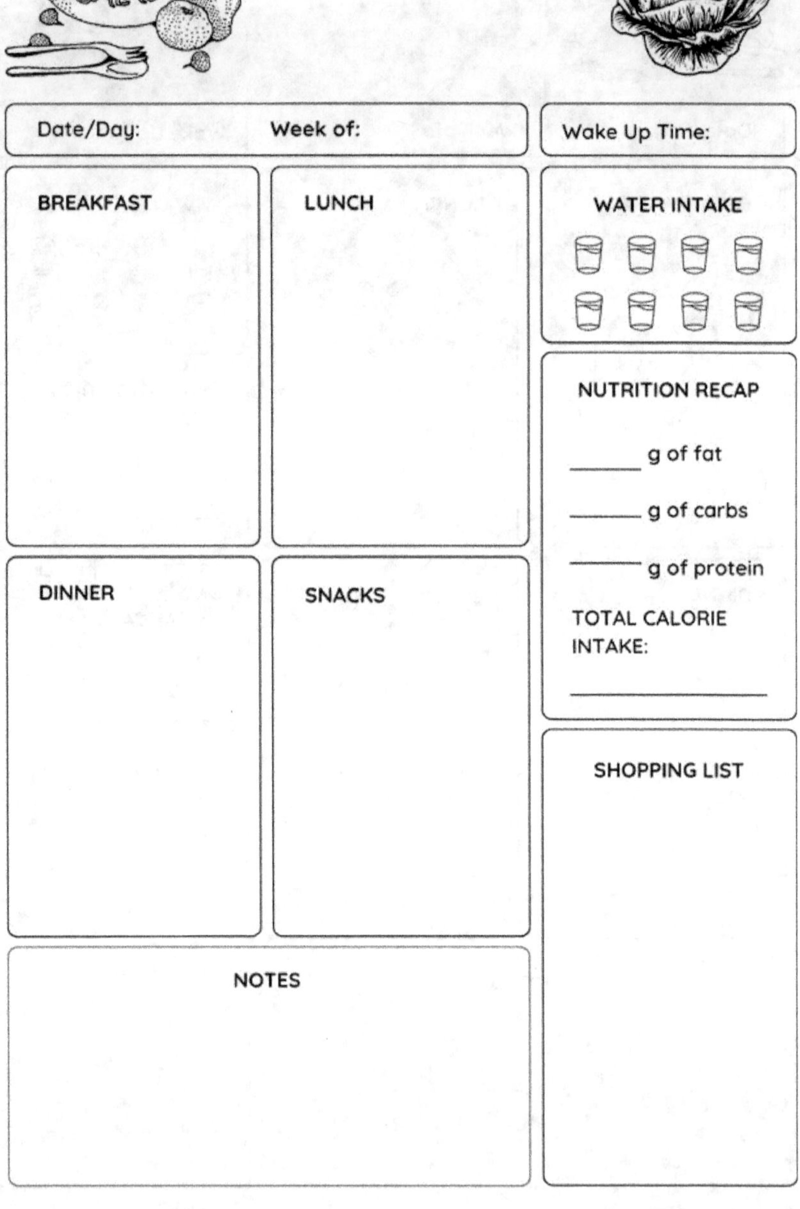

| Date/Day: | Week of: | Wake Up Time: |

BREAKFAST

LUNCH

WATER INTAKE

DINNER

SNACKS

NUTRITION RECAP

_________ g of fat

_________ g of carbs

_________ g of protein

TOTAL CALORIE INTAKE:

____

SHOPPING LIST

NOTES

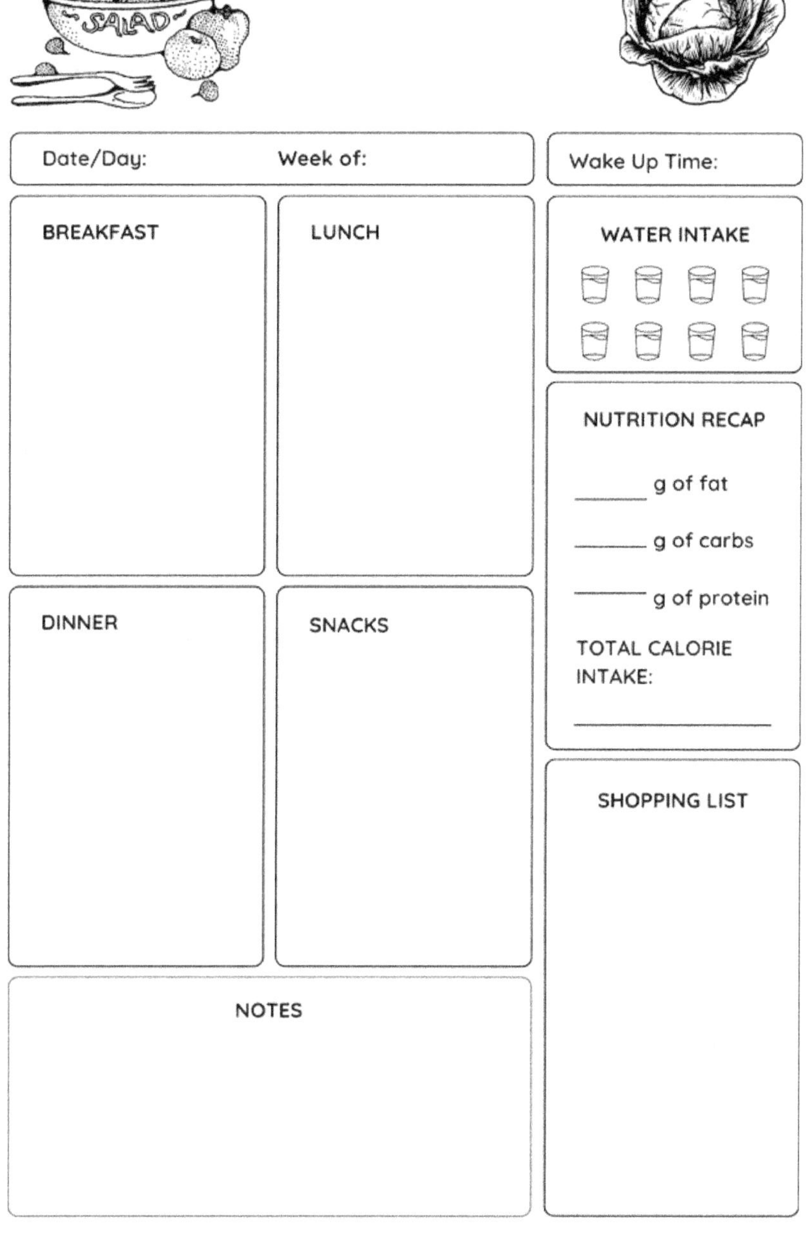

Date/Day:
Week of:
Wake Up Time:
BREAKFAST
LUNCH
WATER INTAKE
NUTRITION RECAP
_______ g of fat
_______ g of carbs
_______ g of protein
TOTAL CALORIE INTAKE:
DINNER
SNACKS
SHOPPING LIST
NOTES

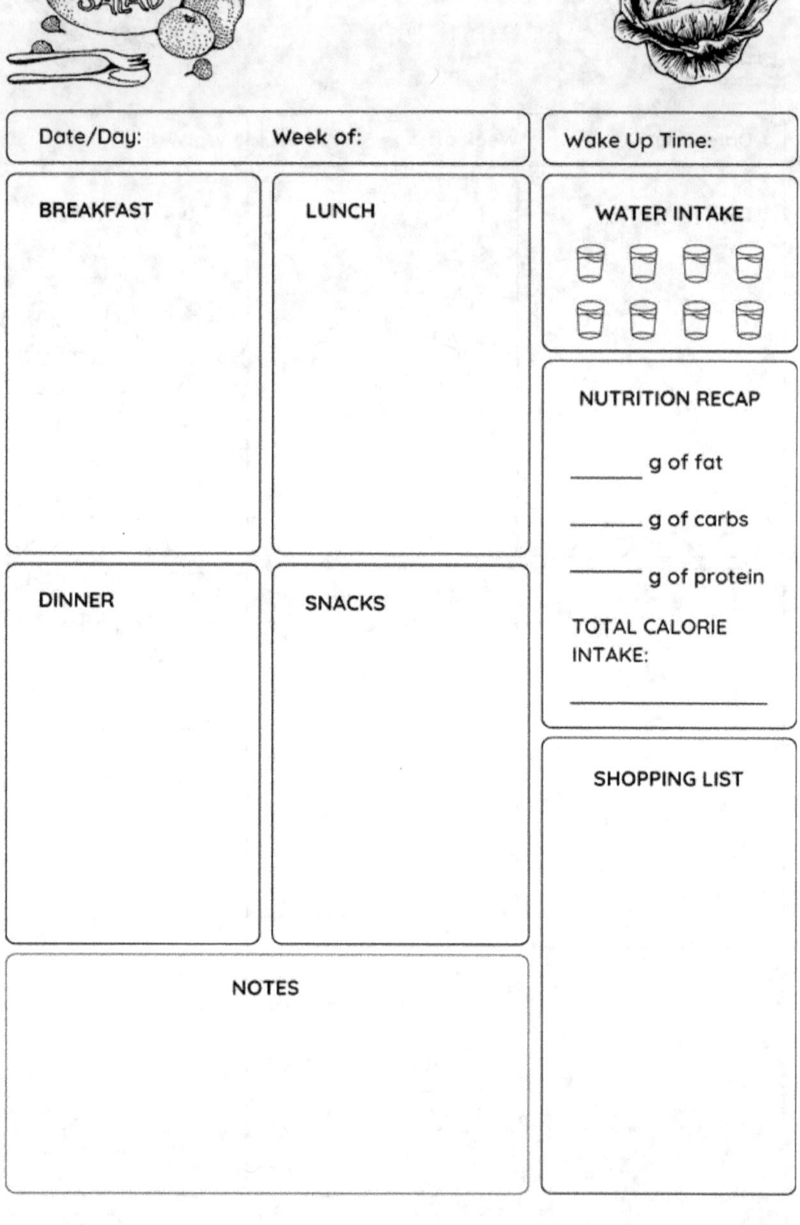

Date/Day: Week of: Wake Up Time:

BREAKFAST

LUNCH

WATER INTAKE

NUTRITION RECAP

_______ g of fat

_______ g of carbs

_______ g of protein

DINNER

SNACKS

TOTAL CALORIE INTAKE:

____

SHOPPING LIST

NOTES

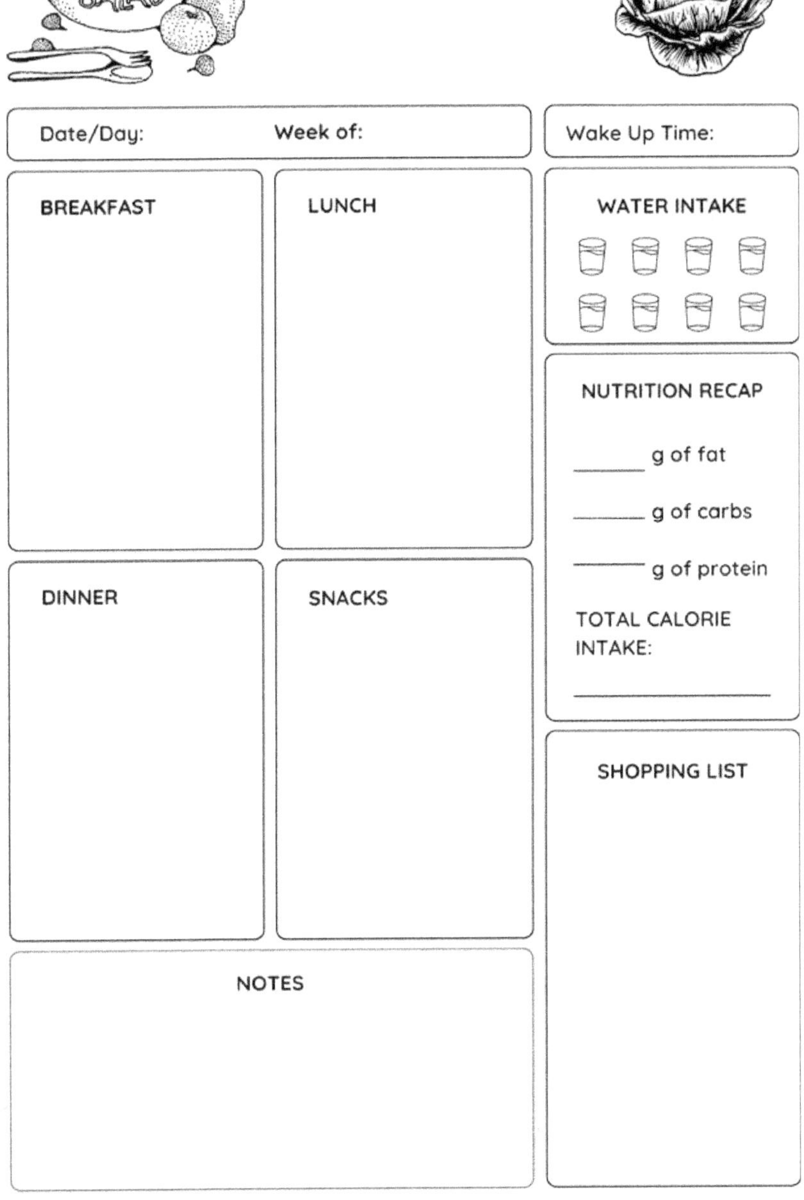

Date/Day: Week of:

Wake Up Time:

BREAKFAST

LUNCH

WATER INTAKE

DINNER

SNACKS

NUTRITION RECAP

_______ g of fat

_______ g of carbs

_______ g of protein

TOTAL CALORIE INTAKE:

____

SHOPPING LIST

NOTES

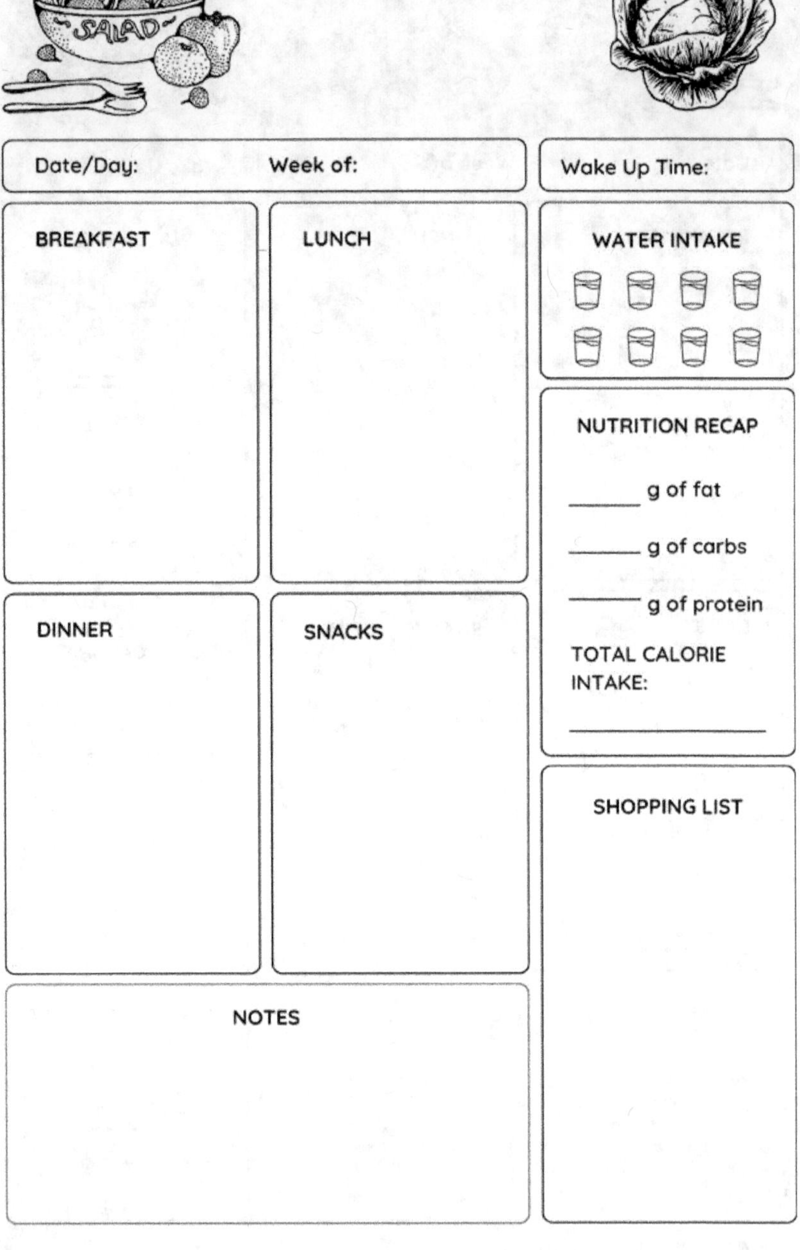

| Date/Day: | Week of: | Wake Up Time: |

BREAKFAST

LUNCH

WATER INTAKE

NUTRITION RECAP

______ g of fat

______ g of carbs

______ g of protein

TOTAL CALORIE INTAKE:

____

DINNER

SNACKS

SHOPPING LIST

NOTES

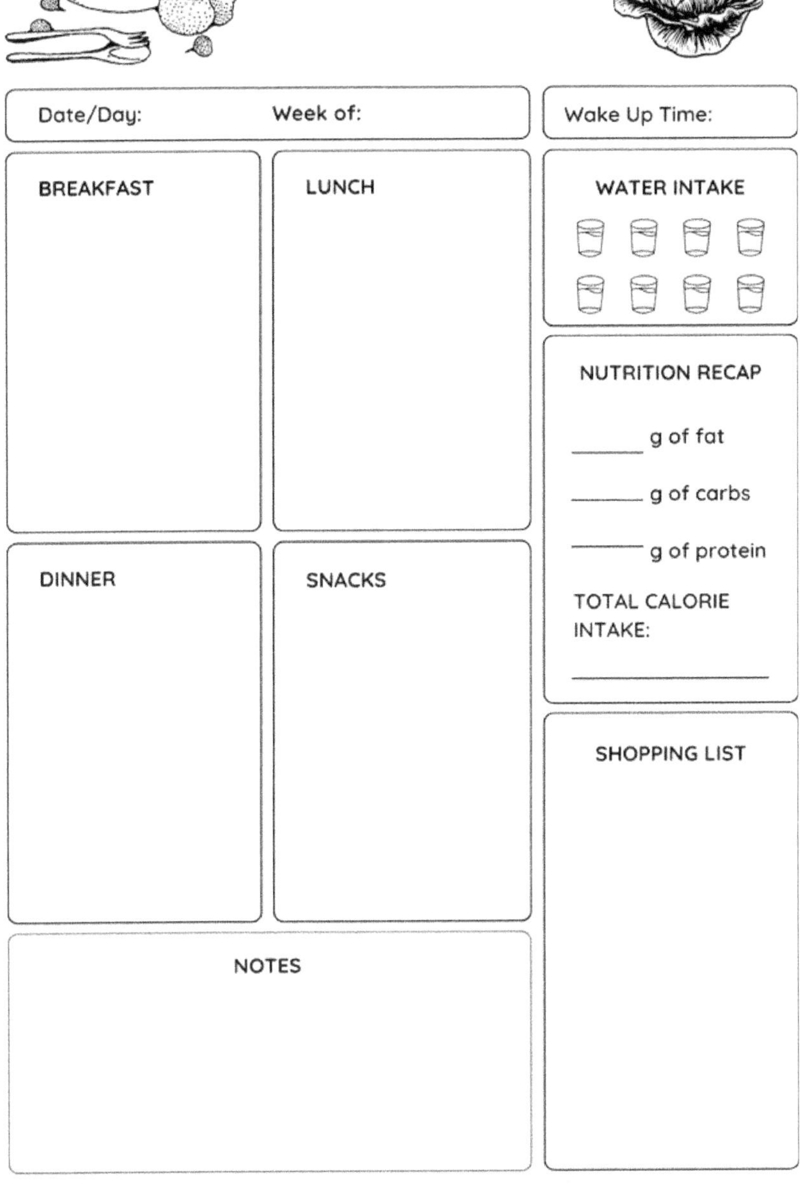

Date/Day: Week of:

Wake Up Time:

BREAKFAST

LUNCH

WATER INTAKE

NUTRITION RECAP

_________ g of fat

_________ g of carbs

_________ g of protein

TOTAL CALORIE INTAKE:

____

DINNER

SNACKS

SHOPPING LIST

NOTES

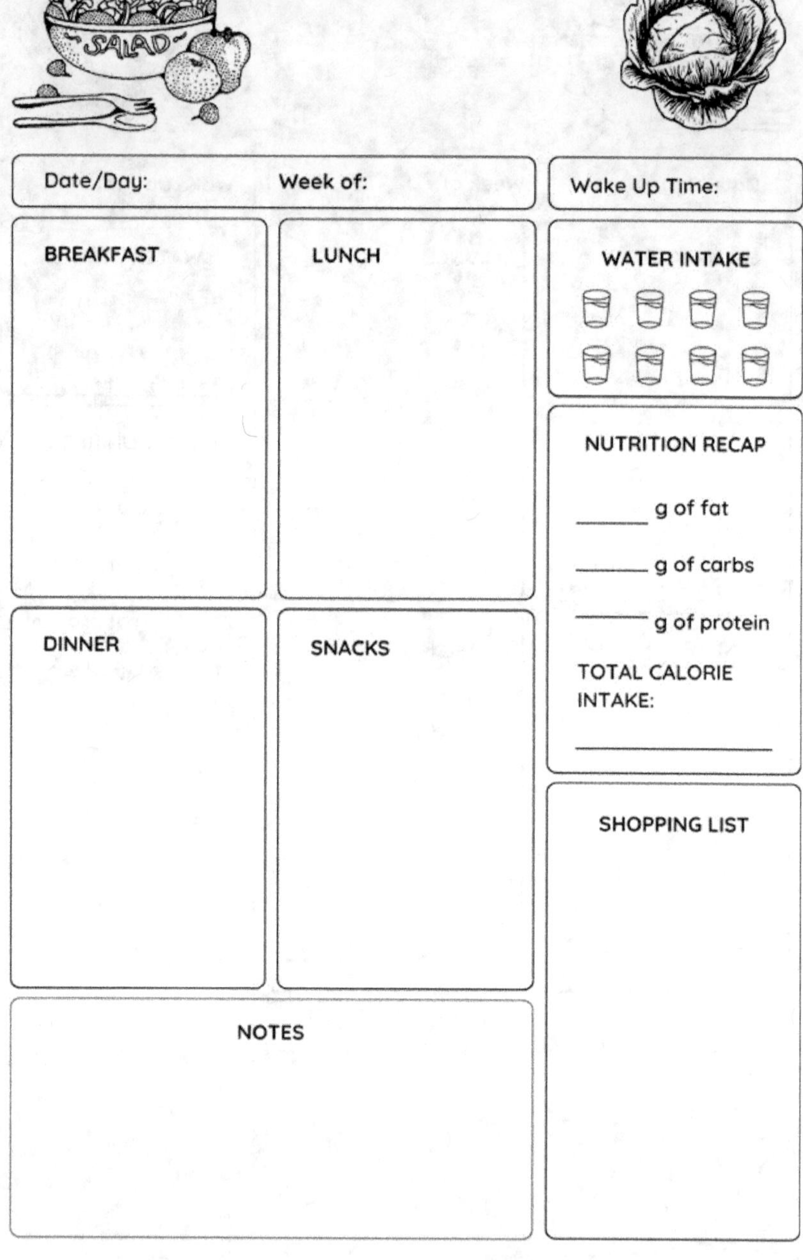

| Date/Day: | Week of: | Wake Up Time: |

BREAKFAST

LUNCH

WATER INTAKE

NUTRITION RECAP

_______ g of fat

_______ g of carbs

_______ g of protein

TOTAL CALORIE INTAKE:

____

DINNER

SNACKS

SHOPPING LIST

NOTES

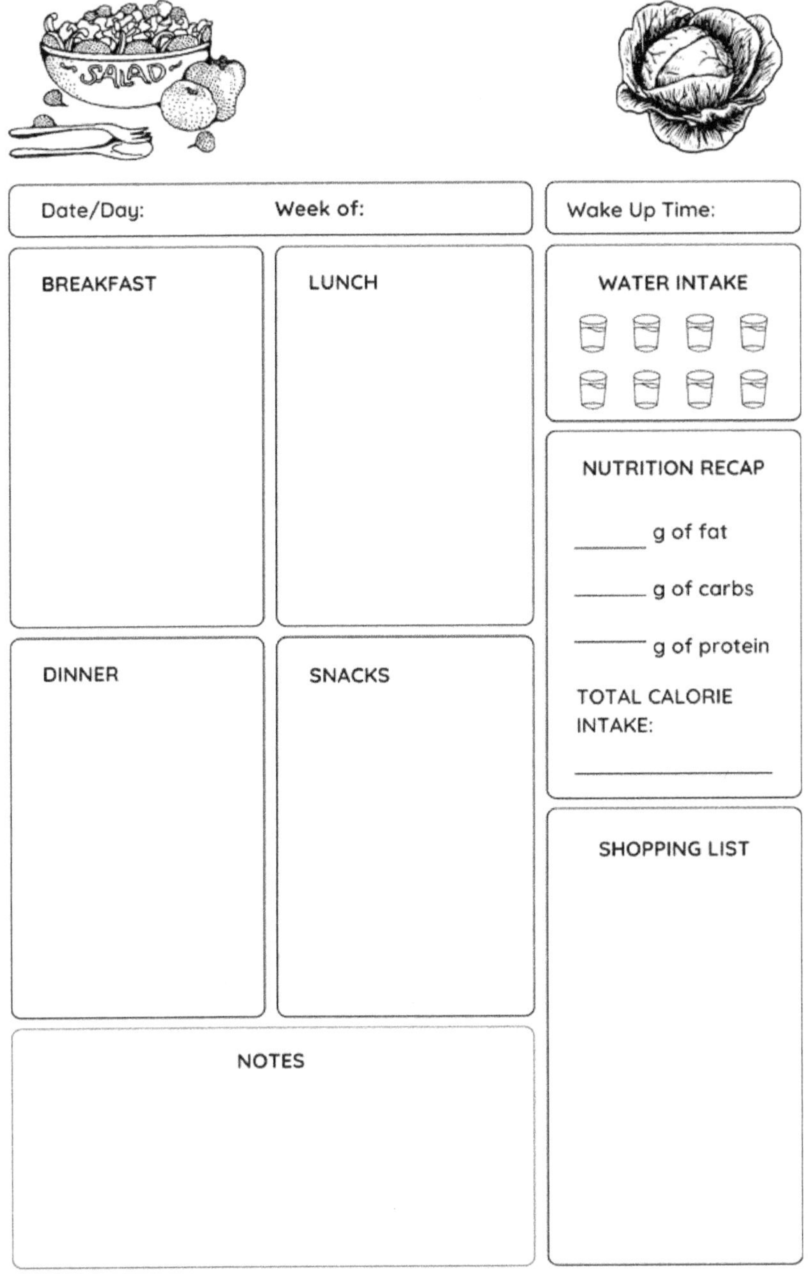

Date/Day:
Week of:
Wake Up Time:
BREAKFAST
LUNCH
WATER INTAKE
NUTRITION RECAP
_______ g of fat
_______ g of carbs
_______ g of protein
TOTAL CALORIE INTAKE:
DINNER
SNACKS
SHOPPING LIST
NOTES

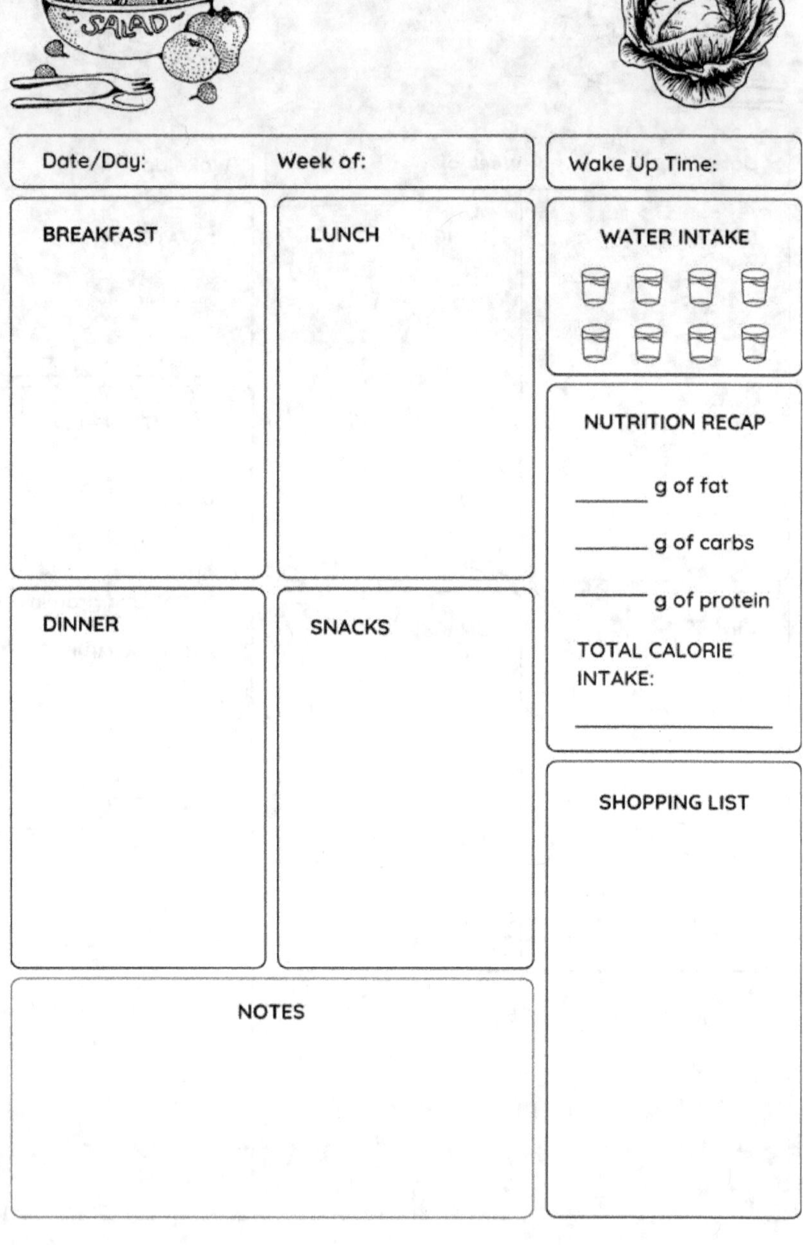

| Date/Day: | Week of: | Wake Up Time: |

BREAKFAST

LUNCH

WATER INTAKE

DINNER

SNACKS

NUTRITION RECAP

_______ g of fat

_______ g of carbs

_______ g of protein

TOTAL CALORIE INTAKE:

SHOPPING LIST

NOTES

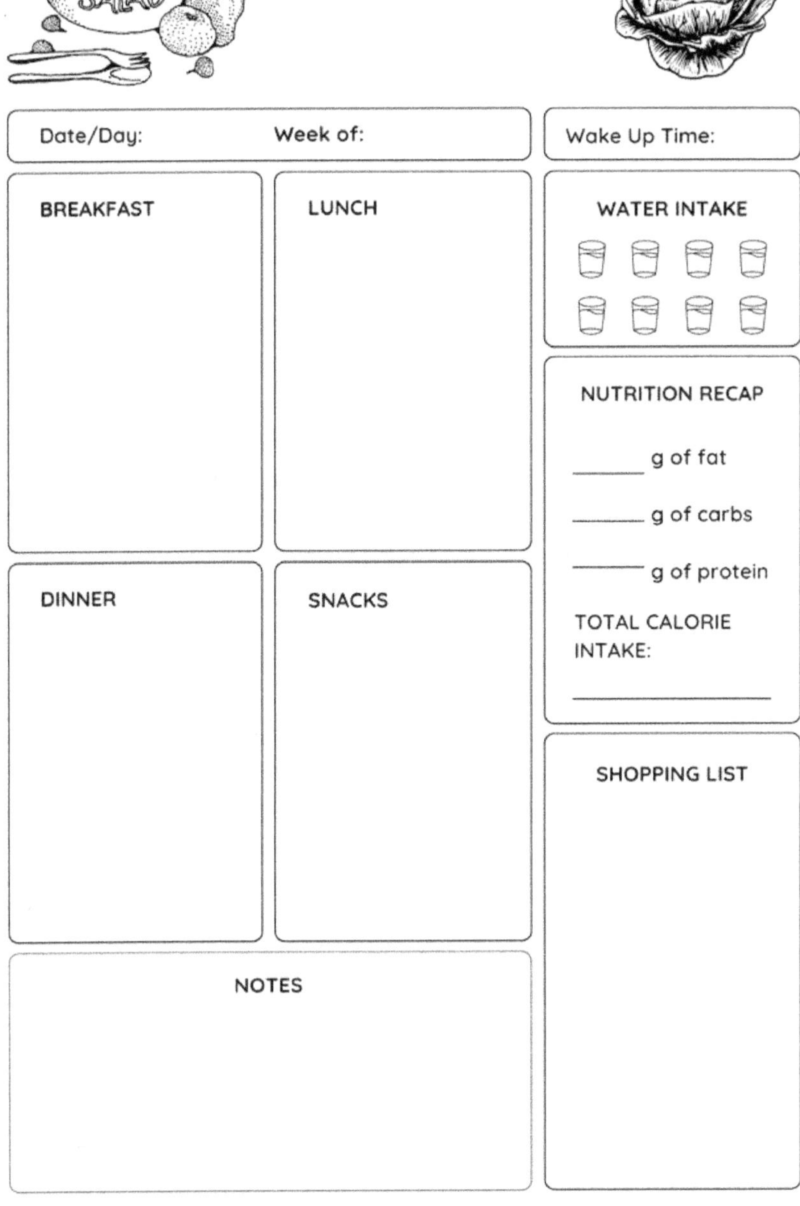

Date/Day: Week of:
Wake Up Time:
BREAKFAST
LUNCH
WATER INTAKE
NUTRITION RECAP
_______ g of fat
_______ g of carbs
_______ g of protein
TOTAL CALORIE INTAKE:
DINNER
SNACKS
SHOPPING LIST
NOTES

Date/Day: | Week of:

Wake Up Time:

BREAKFAST

LUNCH

WATER INTAKE

NUTRITION RECAP

________ g of fat

________ g of carbs

________ g of protein

TOTAL CALORIE INTAKE:

____

DINNER

SNACKS

SHOPPING LIST

NOTES

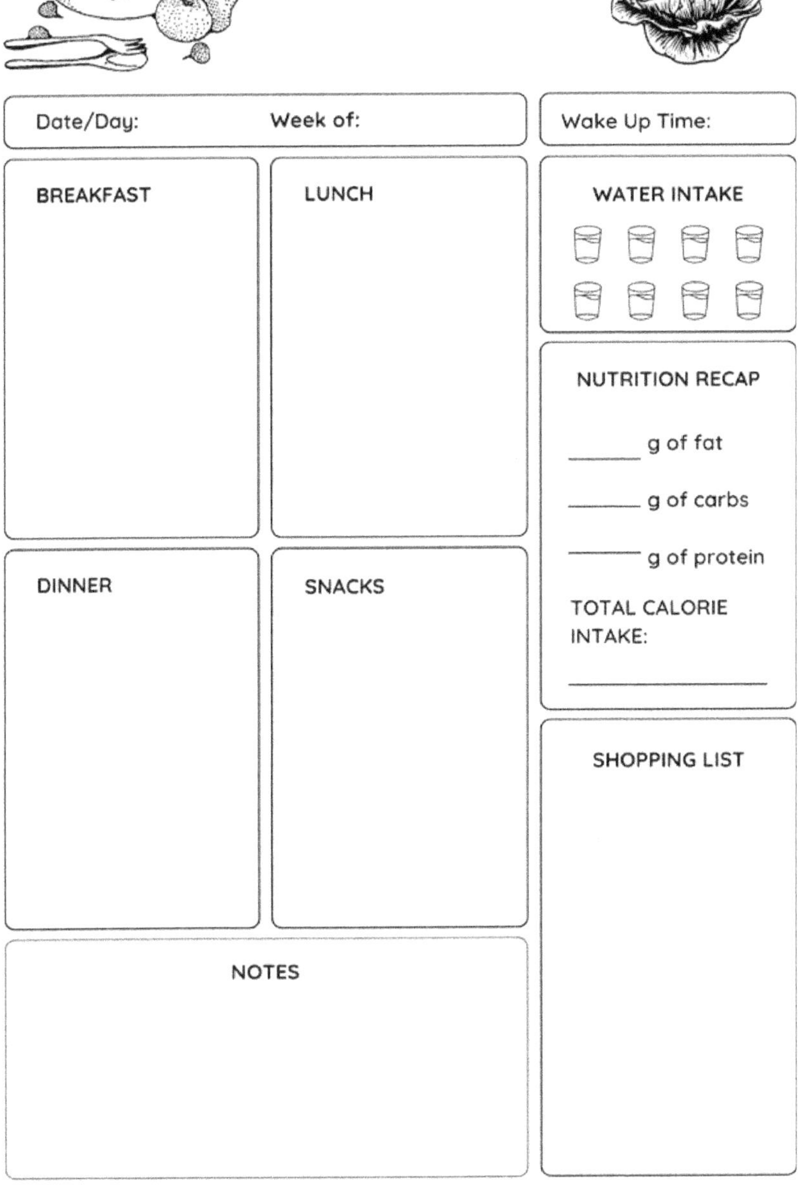

| Date/Day: | Week of: | Wake Up Time: |

BREAKFAST

LUNCH

WATER INTAKE

NUTRITION RECAP

_______ g of fat

_______ g of carbs

_______ g of protein

TOTAL CALORIE INTAKE:

____

DINNER

SNACKS

SHOPPING LIST

NOTES

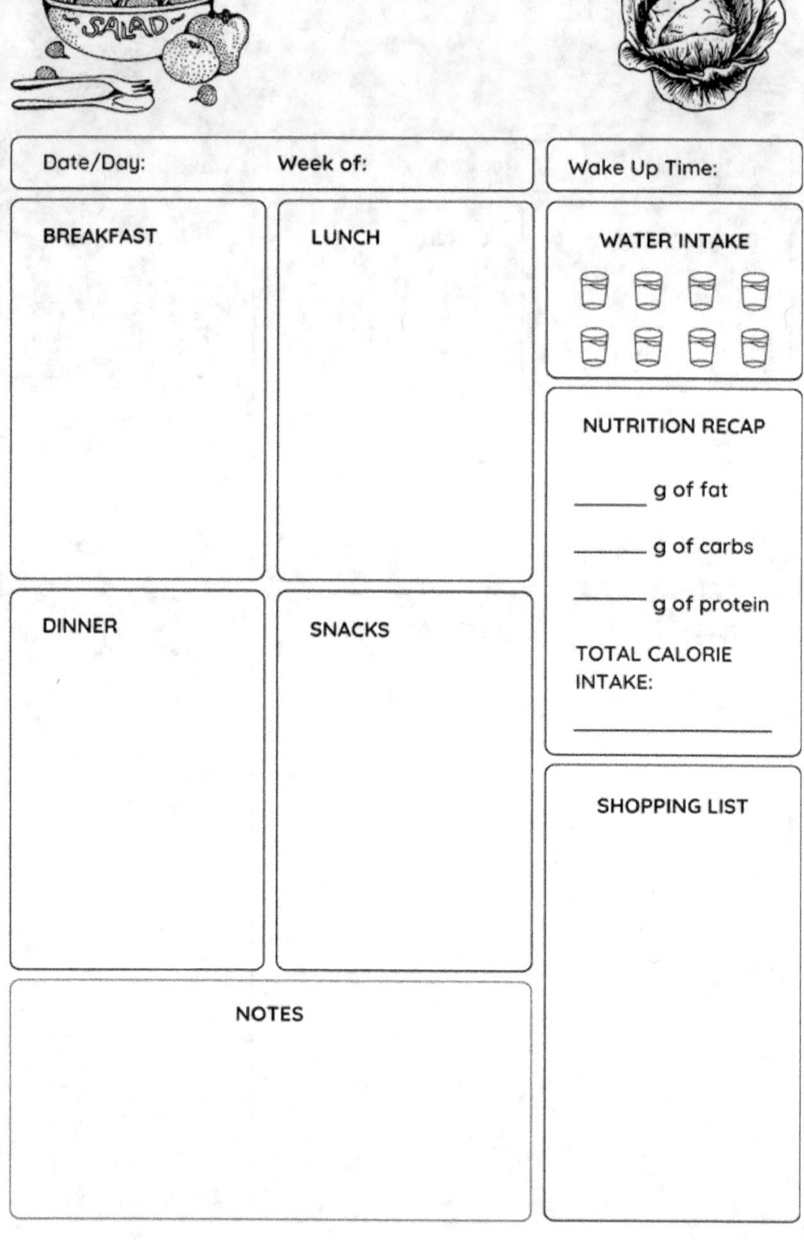

| Date/Day: | Week of: | Wake Up Time: |

BREAKFAST

LUNCH

WATER INTAKE

DINNER

SNACKS

NUTRITION RECAP

_______ g of fat

_______ g of carbs

_______ g of protein

TOTAL CALORIE INTAKE:

____

SHOPPING LIST

NOTES

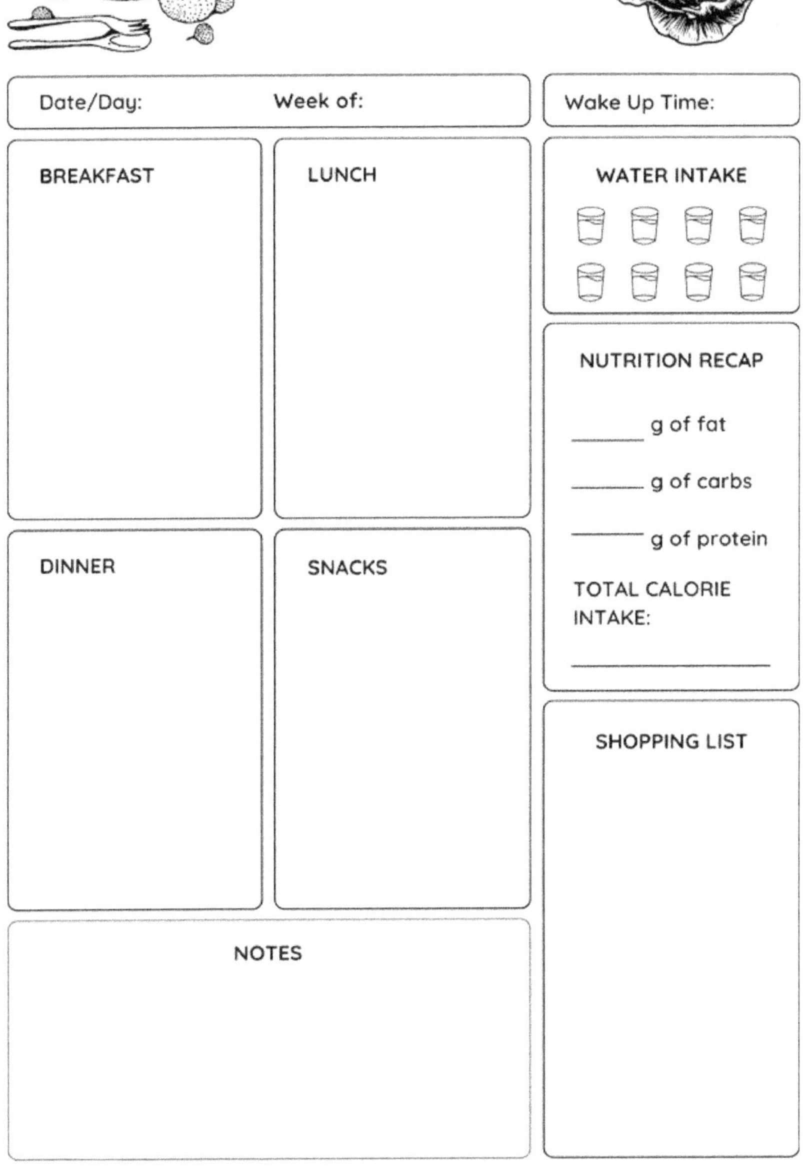

Date/Day:
Week of:
Wake Up Time:
BREAKFAST
LUNCH
WATER INTAKE
NUTRITION RECAP
_______ g of fat
_______ g of carbs
_______ g of protein
TOTAL CALORIE INTAKE:
____
DINNER
SNACKS
SHOPPING LIST
NOTES

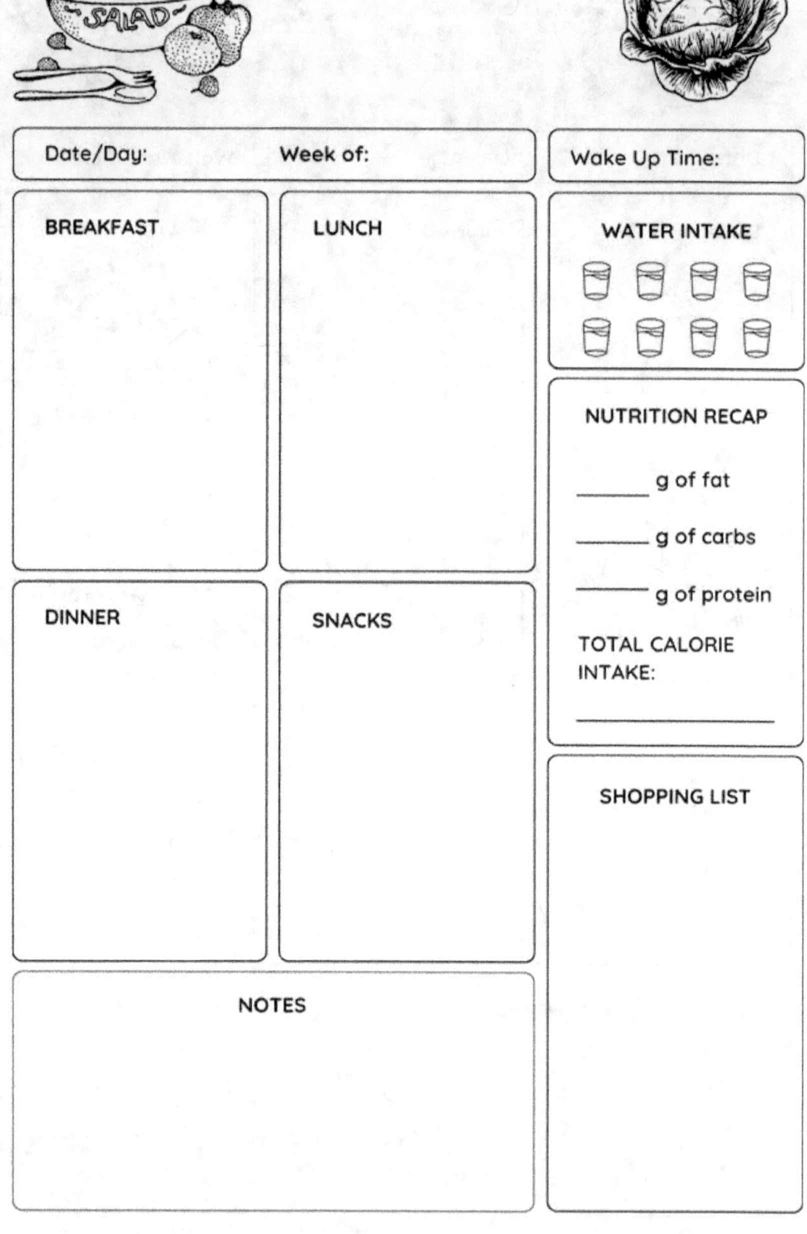

Date/Day:
Week of:
Wake Up Time:
BREAKFAST
LUNCH
WATER INTAKE
NUTRITION RECAP
_______ g of fat
_______ g of carbs
_______ g of protein
TOTAL CALORIE INTAKE:
DINNER
SNACKS
SHOPPING LIST
NOTES

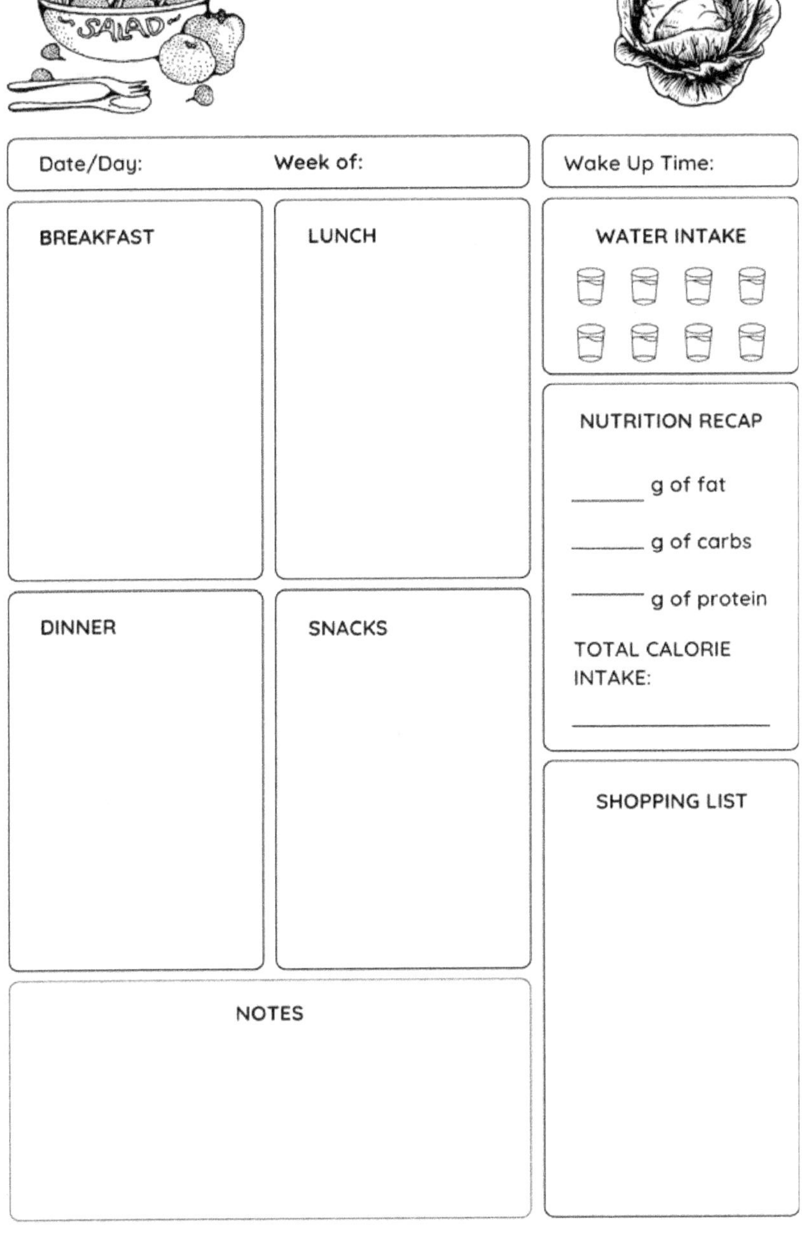

| Date/Day: | Week of: | Wake Up Time: |

BREAKFAST

LUNCH

WATER INTAKE

NUTRITION RECAP

_______ g of fat

_______ g of carbs

_______ g of protein

TOTAL CALORIE INTAKE:

DINNER

SNACKS

SHOPPING LIST

NOTES

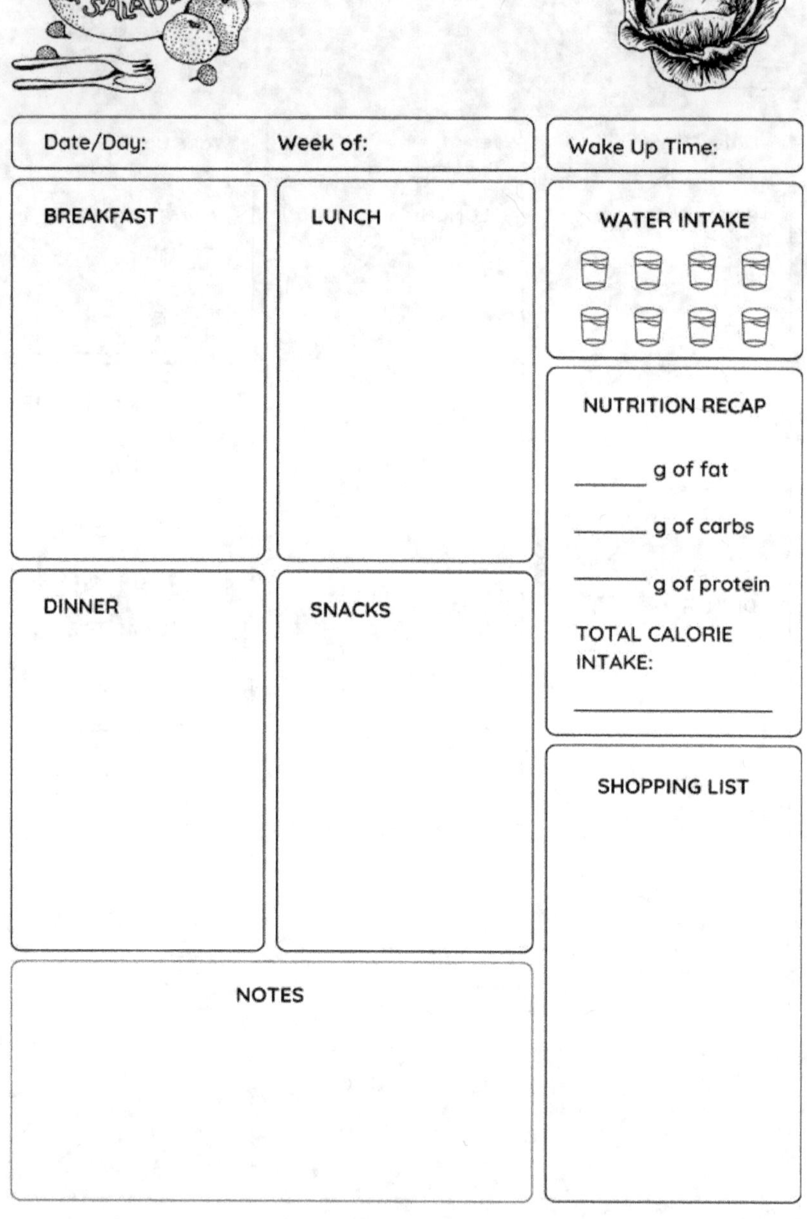

Date/Day:

Week of:

Wake Up Time:

BREAKFAST

LUNCH

WATER INTAKE

NUTRITION RECAP

_______ g of fat

_______ g of carbs

_______ g of protein

TOTAL CALORIE INTAKE:

____

DINNER

SNACKS

SHOPPING LIST

NOTES

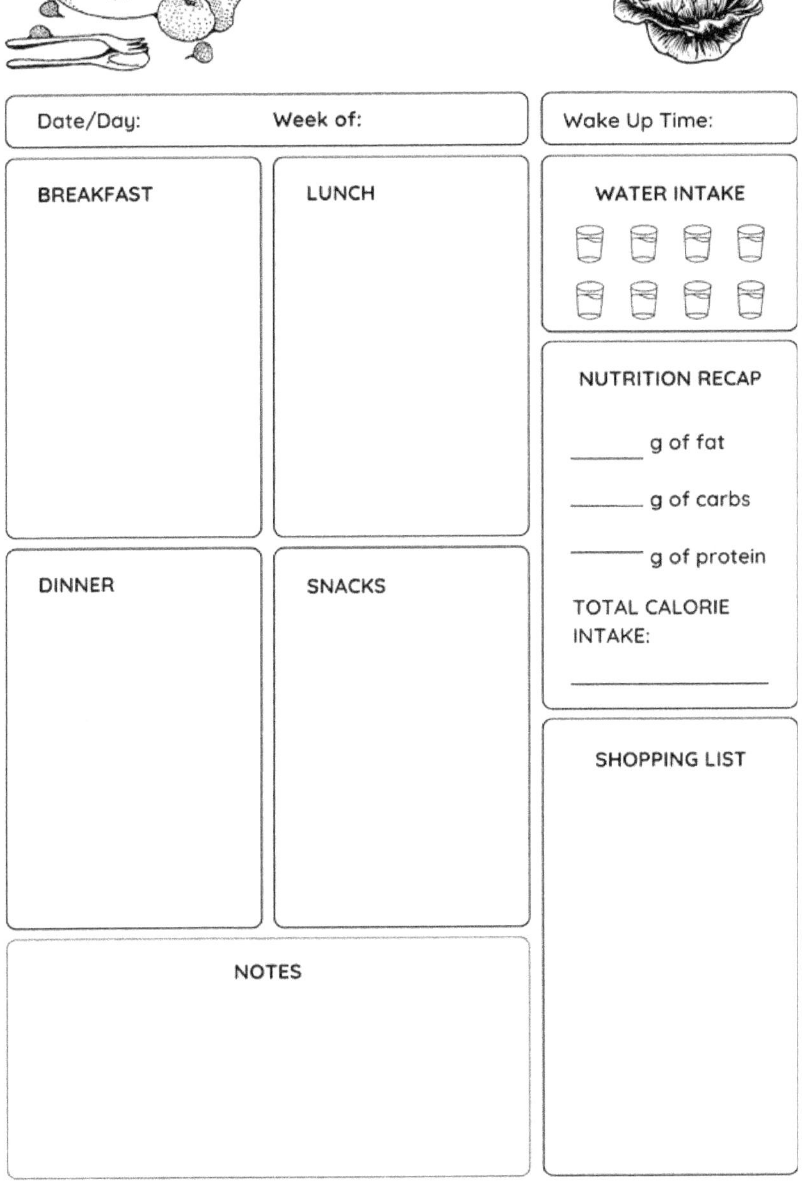

Date/Day: Week of: Wake Up Time:

BREAKFAST

LUNCH

WATER INTAKE

NUTRITION RECAP

_______ g of fat

_______ g of carbs

_______ g of protein

TOTAL CALORIE INTAKE:

DINNER

SNACKS

SHOPPING LIST

NOTES

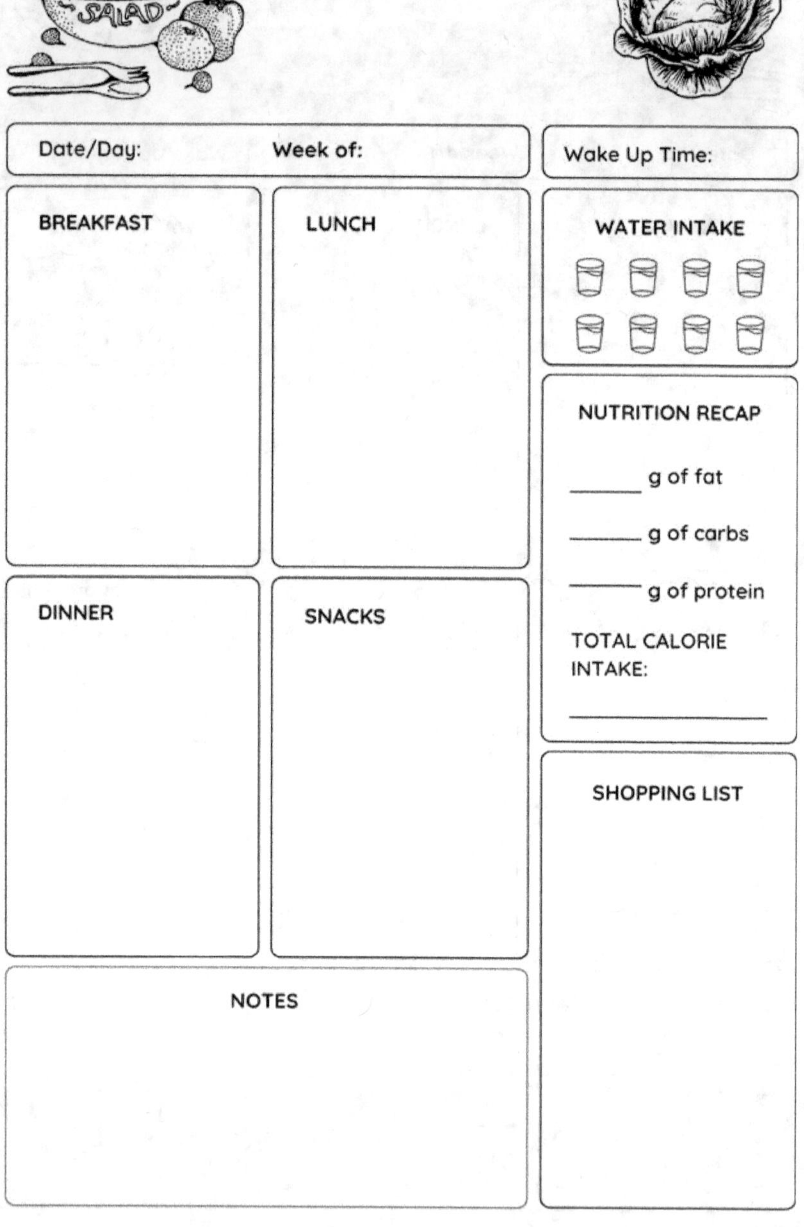

Date/Day: Week of:

Wake Up Time:

BREAKFAST

LUNCH

WATER INTAKE

DINNER

SNACKS

NUTRITION RECAP

_______ g of fat

_______ g of carbs

_______ g of protein

TOTAL CALORIE INTAKE:

____

SHOPPING LIST

NOTES

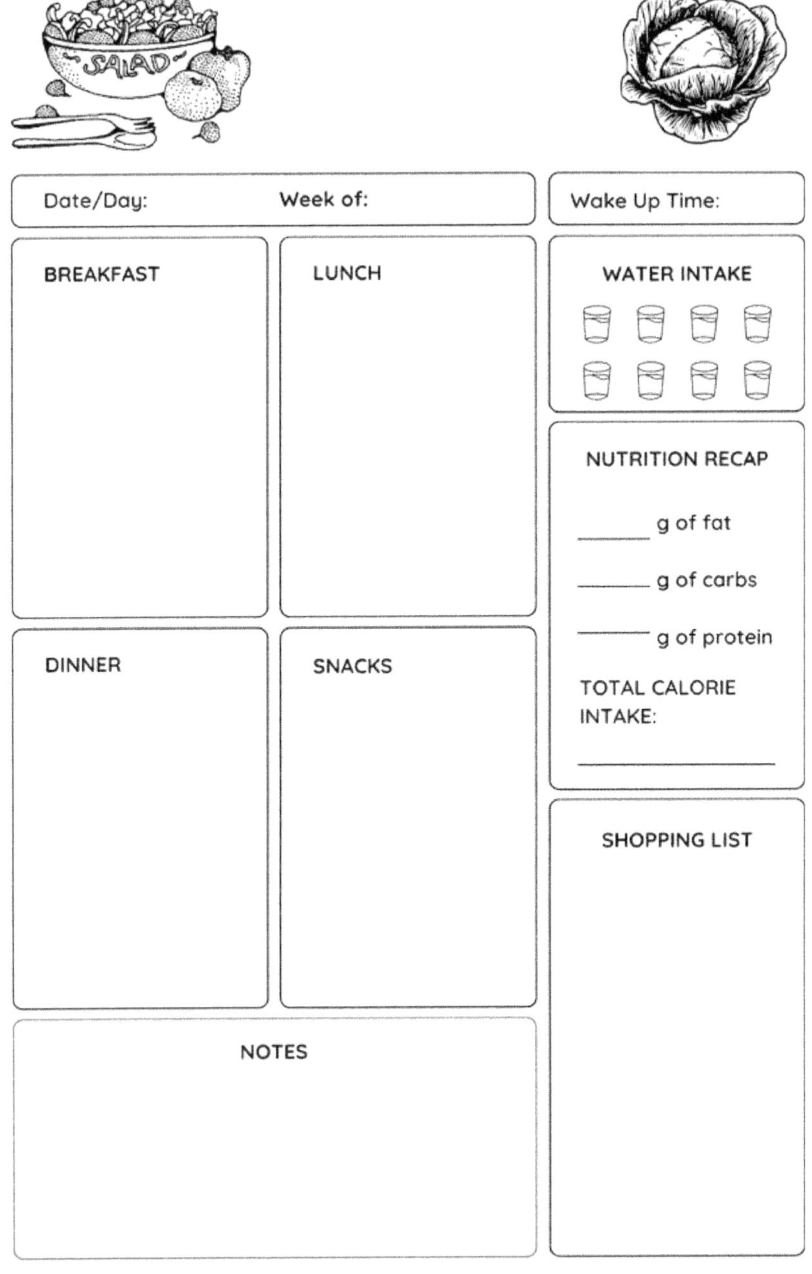

Date/Day:
Week of:
Wake Up Time:
BREAKFAST
LUNCH
WATER INTAKE
NUTRITION RECAP
_______ g of fat
_______ g of carbs
_______ g of protein
TOTAL CALORIE INTAKE:
DINNER
SNACKS
SHOPPING LIST
NOTES

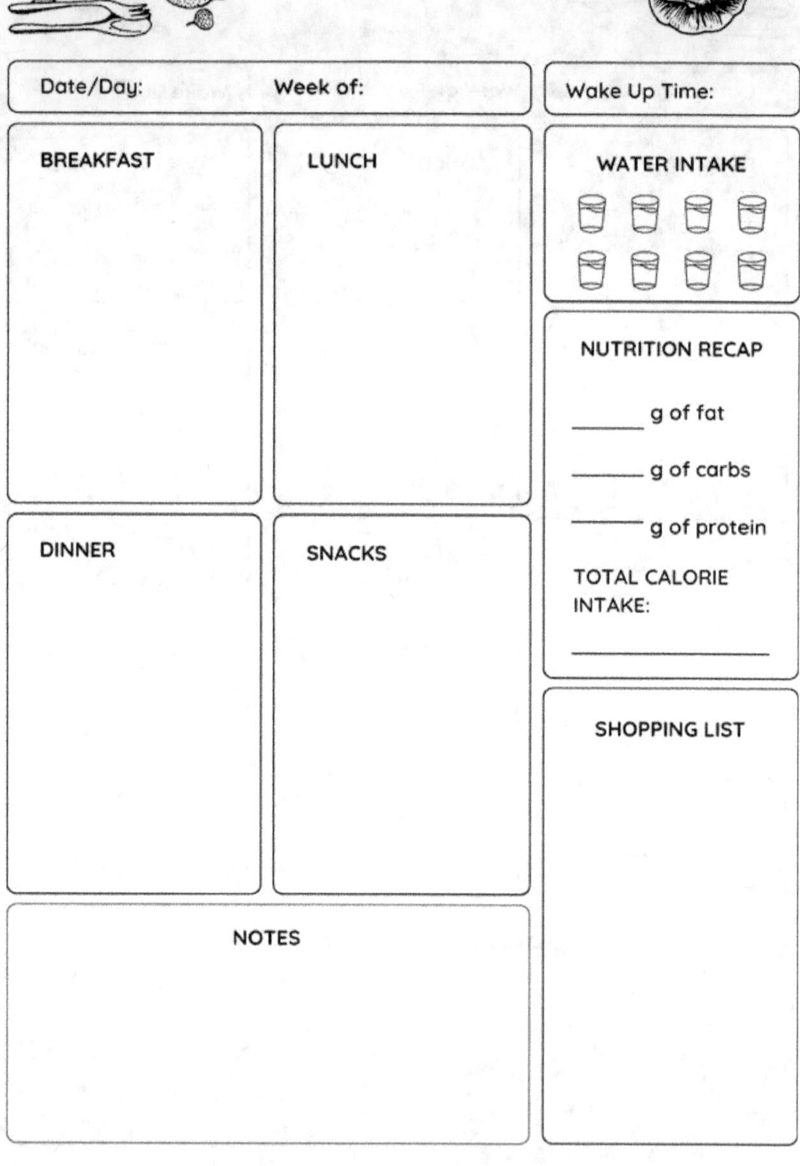

Date/Day: Week of: Wake Up Time:

BREAKFAST

LUNCH

WATER INTAKE

NUTRITION RECAP

_______ g of fat

_______ g of carbs

_______ g of protein

TOTAL CALORIE INTAKE:

____

DINNER

SNACKS

SHOPPING LIST

NOTES